365

nights of passion

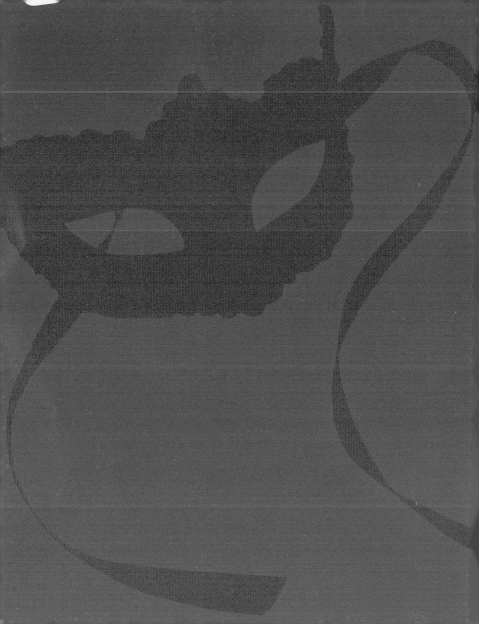

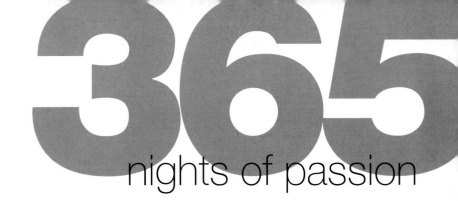

365 nights of passion

London, New York, Melbourne,
Munich, and Delhi

Editor: Louise Frances
Designer: Alison Fenton
Project Editor: Laura Palosuo
Project Art Editor: Katherine Raj
Design Assistant: Laura Mingozzi
Executive Managing Editor: Adèle Hayward
Managing Art Editor: Kat Mead
US Editor: Charles Wills
Production Editor: Kelly Salih
Production Controller: Alice Holloway
Creative Technical Support: Sonia Charbonnier
Art Director: Peter Luff
Publisher: Stephanie Jackson

First American Edition, 2009

Published in the United States by
DK Publishing
375 Hudson Street
New York, New York 10014

09 10 11 12   10 9 8 7 6 5 4 3 2 1

175555—November 2009

Published in Great Britain by Dorling Kindersley Limited.

A catalog record for this book is available from the Library of Congress.

ISBN 978-0-7566-5584-6

DK books are available at special discounts when purchased in bulk for sales promotions, premiums, fund-raising,
or educational use. For details, contact: DK Publishing Special Markets, 375 Hudson Street, New York,
New York 10014 or SpecialSales@dk.com.

Color reproduction by Colourscan, Singapore

Printed and bound in Singapore by Star Standard

Discover more at
www.dk.com

Contents

Introduction

Answer this question before you turn the page:

How's your sex life?

a. comme ci, comme ça
b. up and down, but mostly up
c. totally ooooorgasmic

Whether you answered a, b, or c, this book will pick up your sex life, give it a whole-body shake, and turn it into something spanking new.

This book offers you and your lover 365 nights of amazing sex. By the end of it, you'll have spent nights tying each other up, you'll have tried every possible oral sex position, you'll have had upside-down orgasms, and you'll be a genius with sex toys. You may also have woken up dressed as a milkmaid.

Nights of no-frills missionary will be a distant memory.

Yes, there'll be hazards along the way... You may think "we didn't really do THAT last night, did we?" You may get envious looks from your neighbors. Your mattress may never be the same again.

But, follow these simple passion precautions, and you'll have the best year of your life:

● If you're pushing your partner's kink boundaries, be nice and respectful. Ask them to shout a safeword if they get to the "get me out of here" stage.

● Be precious about hygiene— if something (meaning a penis/ dildo/phallic-shaped vegetable) goes in or around the anus, it mustn't go anywhere near her vagina afterward. To put it another way, you can have vaginal sex followed by anal sex, but don't do it the other way round.

● Don't break the law. You may adore al fresco sex on hotel balconies—the local police may not. The same applies to swimming-pool, gym, and elevator sex—don't perform to an audience. Or, if you HAVE to perform to an audience, rent a private mansion and throw a fantastically debauched party.

● When attempting a backward flip or hanging off the ceiling, always make sure you've got something soft to land on.

Now slip into something comfortable and turn the page. Whether you want to make amour like an angel, canoodle like a cat, or tussle like a tiger, you'll find a night to bring you bliss. Remember: it's one thing to share a week of passion with your lover, another thing to share a month of passion, but...

To share a YEAR of passion will secure you a lifetime achievement award for sexual service. Enjoy the romp.

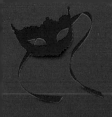

Perfect for pure romance

Try these when you want to swoon:

Perfect for a sexy workout

Try these when you want to feel stretched:

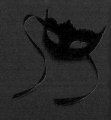

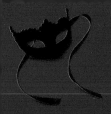

Perfect for rampant naughtiness

Try these when you want to be wicked:

Perfect for giggling on the job

Try these when you want light-hearted passion:

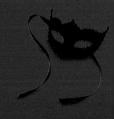

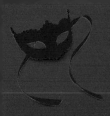

Perfect for fast, hot sex

Try these when you want each other RIGHT NOW:

Perfect for pushing your boundaries

Try these when you want something sexy and novel:

1 Tickling his fancy

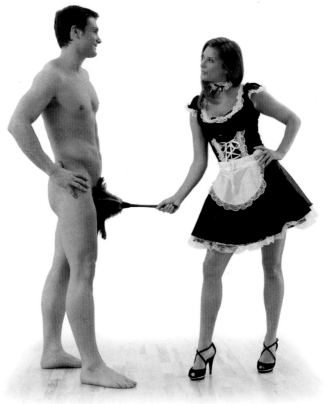

Tonight: She makes it her business to feather him into a fervor.

Quickie passion: She offers him a slick, wet polish.
Lingering passion: She asks him to lie back for the deluxe maid service.

Erotic Olympics 2

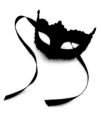

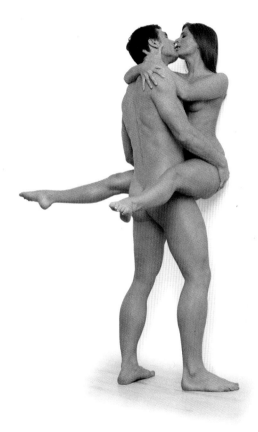

Tonight: You go for gold in a mind-blowing positionathon.

Beginner passion: She delivers a star performance on his bar.
Sexpert passion: You turn your bedroom into a naughty sexy gym.

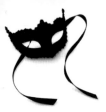

3 Animal passion

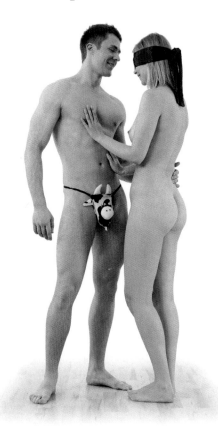

Tonight: He blindfolds her, and he invites her to explore his animal side.

Sweet passion: You swap roles, and he pulls her close, and grazes on her skin.
Wild passion: She rips off his undies to feel the beast beneath.

Playing rampant rabbit 4

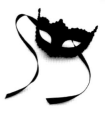

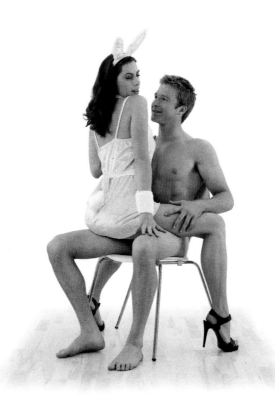

Tonight: She hops on to his lap, and spends the evening as his favorite pet.

Sweet passion: He strokes her adoringly, and tells her how cute she is.
Wild passion: He plunges eagerly into her warren.

5 Thrill sergeant

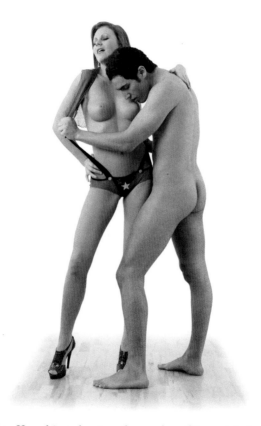

Tonight: He subjects her to a thorough, military-style inspection.

Clean passion: He gives her precision-targeted kisses on both breasts.
Kinky passion: He orders her to do a set of naked push-ups.

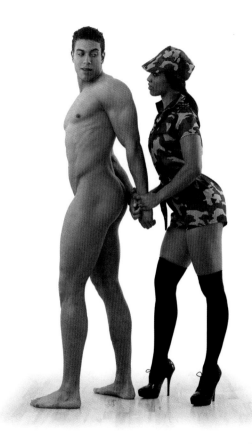

Tonight: She plays the horny GI out to capture him.

Clean passion: She skillfully deploys his heavy weapon.
Kinky passion: She takes him prisoner, and ties him up.

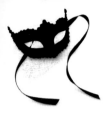

7 Sex on the beach

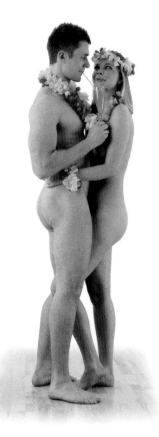

Tonight: You enjoy an evening of fruity cocktails and sexy holiday stories.

Fun passion: He feeds his juicy cocktail cherry to her.
Fervent passion: You dance steamily to hot beach music.

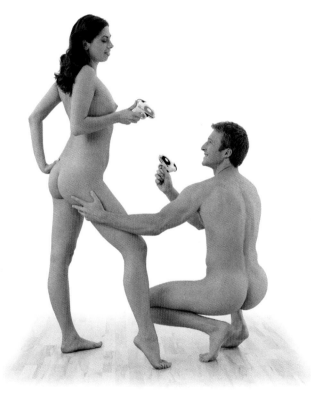

Tonight: You arm yourselves with water pistols, and battle it out in the buff.

Sweet passion: You warm the water first.
Wild passion: You run whooping and yelling around the yard.

9 Tasting session

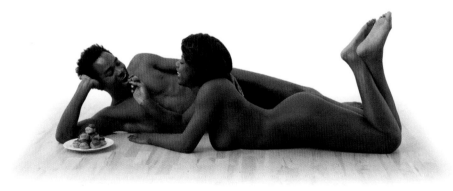

Tonight: She supplies him with endless tasty treats.

Fun passion: She shows him her tongue-twirling and cream-sucking skills.
Fervent passion: She feeds him sweet morsels with her mouth.

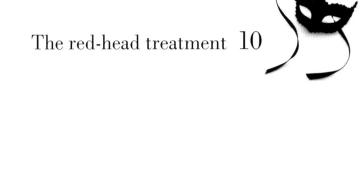

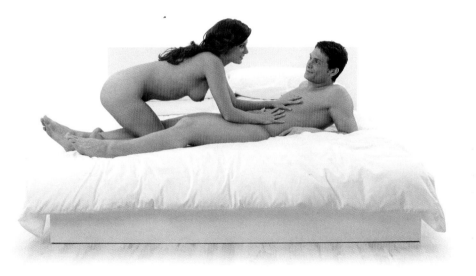

Tonight: She gives him the red-headed vixen experience.

Beginner passion: She relies on a red wig to inflame him.
Sexpert passion: She wears a red wig and a shamelessly seductive corset.

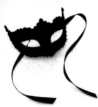

11 Gangster paradise

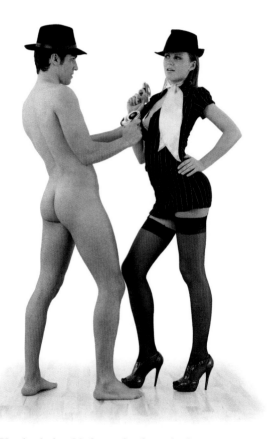

Tonight: You both don Mafia outfits for a shady gangster stand-off.

Beginner passion: She invites him to check out her underworld.
Sexpert passion: She takes off her pinstripes in a pro-style striptease.

Horny devil 12

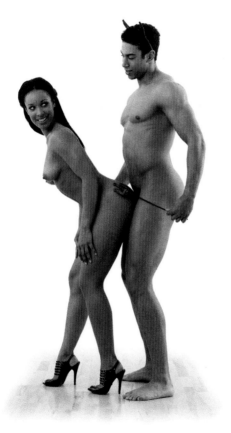

Tonight: He leads her into temptation with wicked strokes of his trident.

Sweet passion: She kisses him, and tells him that he's a handsome devil.
Wild passion: She takes him by the horns, and squeezes his trident.

13 Fruity frolics

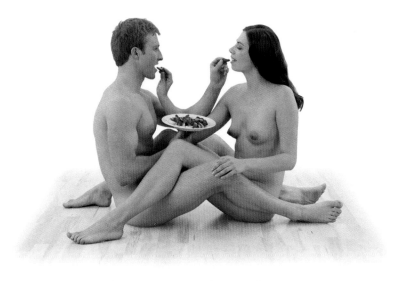

Tonight: You choose some exotic fruits, and start on a juicy note.

Fun passion: You smear each other with fruit, and romp messily.
Fervent passion: He slides a succulent berry into her mouth with each kiss.

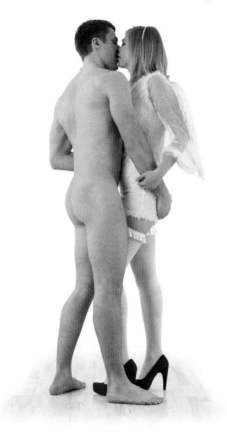

Tonight: She puts on her angel wings, and plays the heavenly innocent.

Quickie passion: He corrupts her with just one kiss.
Lingering passion: She keeps her halo intact nearly all night.

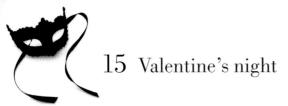

15 Valentine's night

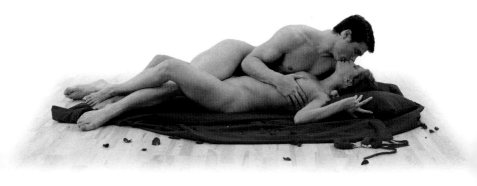

Tonight: She makes him go red on the most romantic night of the year.

Sweet passion: She says a breathy, "I love you."
Wild passion: He handcuffs her, and makes her truly his.

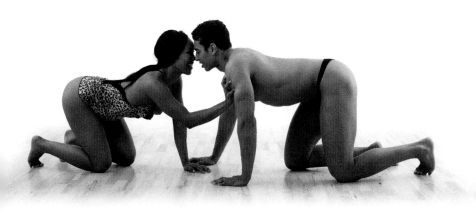

Tonight: You slip into sexy cat costumes, and circle each other hungrily.

Clean passion: You lick each other into lustful oblivion.
Kinky passion: You release your bad tiger: claw, bite, snarl, and pounce.

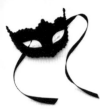

17 Saucy striptease

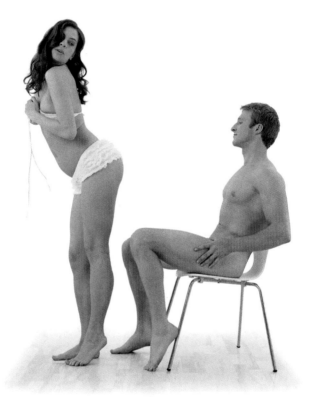

Tonight: She puts on a show that makes him rigid with desire.

Beginner passion: She slides her panties slowly down her thighs.
Sexpert passion: She follows up with an explosive lap dance.

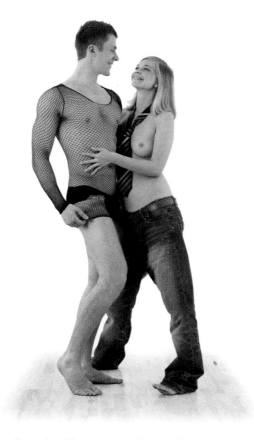

Tonight: She turns macho, and he goes girly.

Fun passion: You give each other new names.
Fervent passion: You surrender joyously to a night of S&D.

19 Charming the pants off her

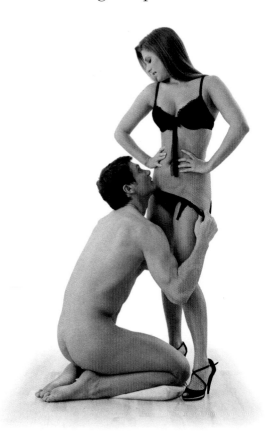

Tonight: He uses all his seductive powers to get inside her pants.

Clean passion: He acts the courteous gentleman throughout.
Kinky passion: He turns tiger, and tears her undies off with his teeth.

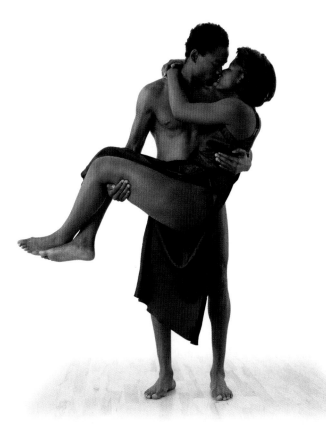

Tonight: She's so irresistible that he grabs her, and carries her off to bed.

Sweet passion: He gives her mouth-melting kisses on the way.
Wild passion: He throws her on to the bed, and jumps on top of her.

21 Erotic Truth or Dare

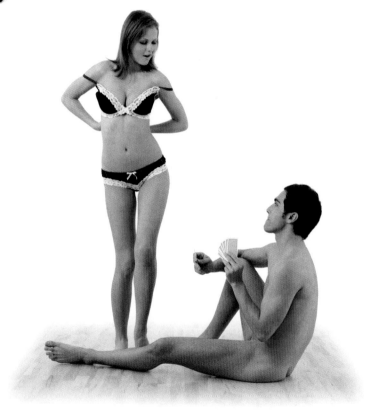

Tonight: You throw yourselves into a naughty evening of Truth or Dare.

Beginner's passion: Agree the questions and dares before you start.
Sexpert passion: You make it as kinky as possible, and ask a friend to join you.

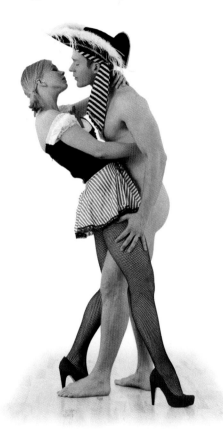

Tonight: He shivers her timbers with raunchy pirate sex.

Sweet passion: He caresses her booty, and shares his rum with her.
Wild passion: He sweeps her off her feet, and pierces her with his mast.

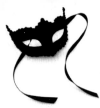

23 Getting down on the ranch

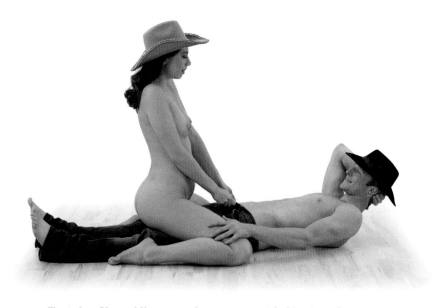

Tonight: She saddles up, and prepares to ride him into the sunset.

Quickie passion: She kicks her heels, and goes rodeo on him.
Lingering passion: She rocks him gently up on to the high plains.

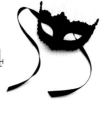

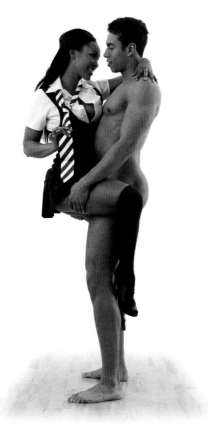

Tonight: She plays the sizzling schoolgirl that he just has to seduce.

Sweet passion: She whispers that she forgot to wear panties.
Wild passion: He presses her against a wall, and goes hell for leather.

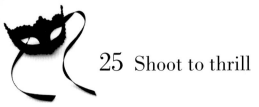

25 Shoot to thrill

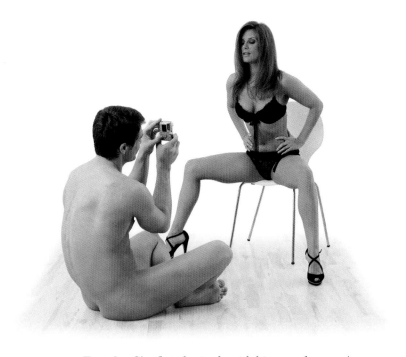

Tonight: She flirts brazenly with his zoom lens.

Fun passion: He uses the self-timer, and joins her in a sexy pose.

Fervent passion: She gets high on revealing one naughty bit at a time.

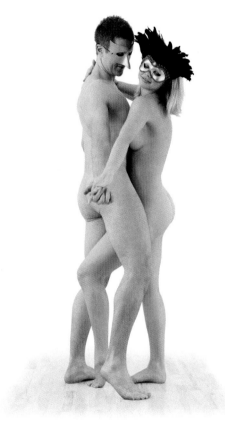

Tonight: You stage a private candlelit ball. Dress code: masks only.

Clean passion: You push your masks back to enjoy a kiss.
Kinky passion: You're silent strangers all night—even during sex.

27 Show and thrill

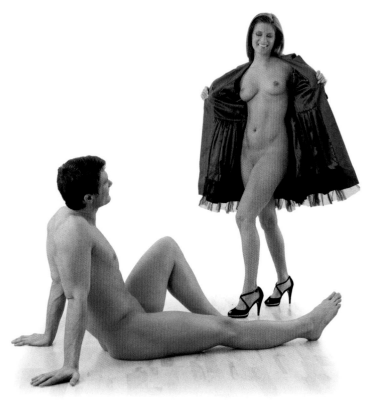

Tonight: She's his horny stranger who can't help flashing her bits.

Beginner passion: She asks him to help her off with her coat.
Sexpert passion: She shimmies off her coat, and does an erotic dance.

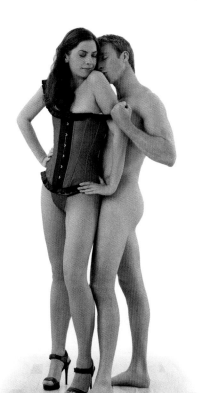

Tonight: She's his birthday treat—all he has to do is unwrap her.

Clean passion: She offers him a sensual birthday massage.
Kinky passion: She'll be his sluttish sex slave for one night only.

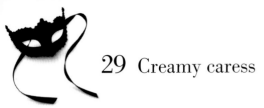

29 Creamy caress

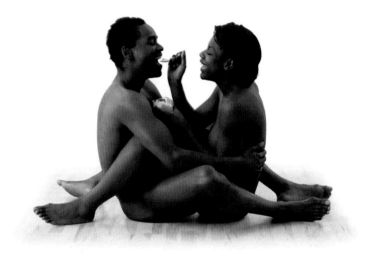

Tonight: You snuggle up in bed, and feed each other velvety, soft ice cream.

Fun passion: She drips ice cream on his lickable bits.
Fervent passion: You drop the ice cream in your haste to get to each other.

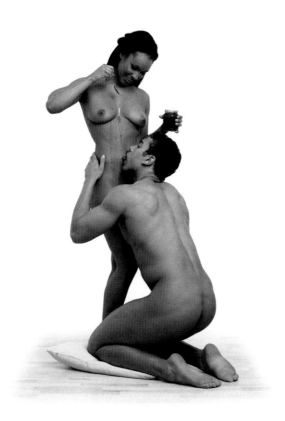

Tonight: She tempts him with something sweet and sticky.

Quickie passion: He makes a beeline for the source of her nectar.
Lingering passion: He slowly licks every last drop of honey from her skin.

31 The art of undressing

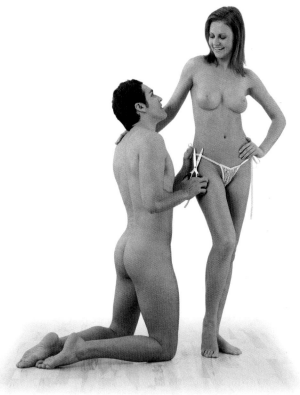

Tonight: He uses all means to get into her pants—hands, teeth, scissors.

Sweet passion: He presents her with some sexy new undies the next night.
Wild passion: He stays on his knees, and ravishes her with his tongue.

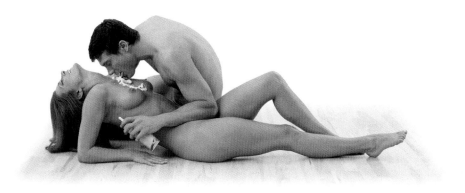

Tonight: He smothers her in whipped cream, and eats her all up.

Quickie passion: He slides his milk machine smoothly inside her.
Lingering passion: He draws creamy patterns all over her body.

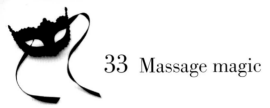

33 Massage magic

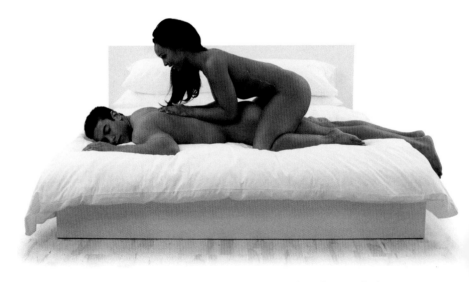

Tonight: She lays him down in her steamy parlor, then works her magic.

Beginner passion: She uses her hands and hair to make him shiver.
Sexpert passion: She uses her hard nipples to make him tremble.

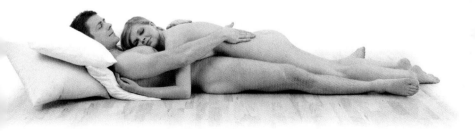

Tonight: He gets her tingling with soft strokes as she lies in his arms.

Fun passion: The more he pets her, the more she purrs.
Fervent passion: You breathe in harmony as the mood heats up.

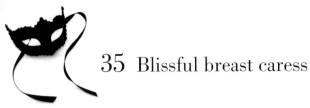

35 Blissful breast caress

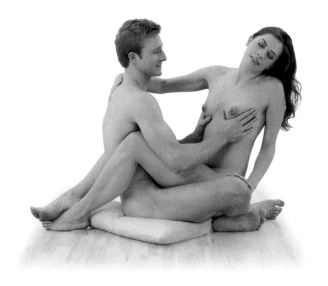

Tonight: He gives his undivided attention to her assets.

Clean passion: He strokes his palms across the whole of her chest.
Kinky passion: He nips her nipples until she cries out with pleasure.

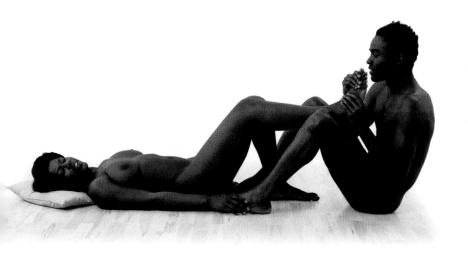

Tonight: He discovers the way to her pleasure palace is through her feet.

Beginner passion: He pushes his oiled fingers in and out between her toes.
Sexpert passion: He takes her toes in his mouth, and sucks them hard.

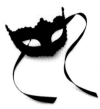

37 Cheeky cheek rub

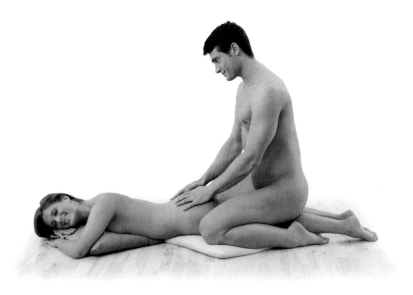

Tonight: He slides his hot hands over her gorgeous mounds.

Quickie passion: She opens her legs in a horny invitation.
Lingering passion: He plays the strictly professional masseuse.

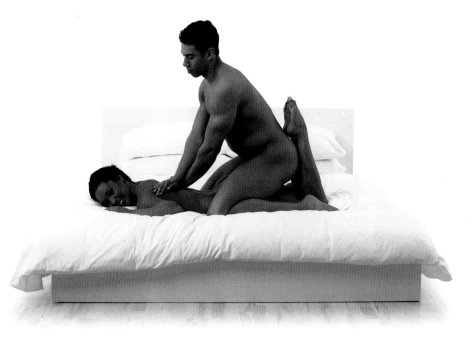

Tonight: You give each other a massage: he uses hands; she uses feet.

Fun passion: She wears furry mittens on her feet.
Fervent passion: He uses the massage tool that's sprung up between his legs.

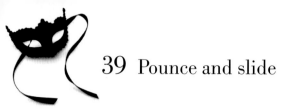

39 Pounce and slide

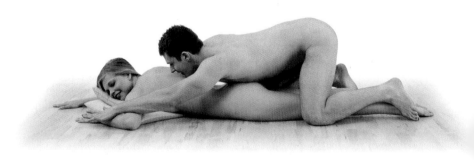

Tonight: He starts at her feet, and gives her body a swooping massage.

Sweet passion: He coats her in massage oil so that he slides smoothly.
Wild passion: He makes her soar by slamming his horn into her.

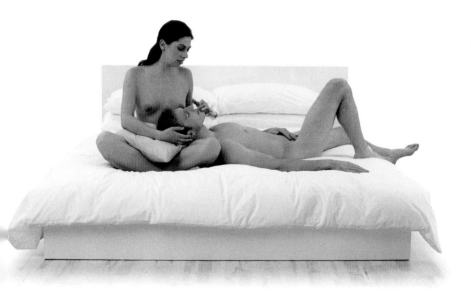

Tonight: She makes his whole body tingle with her fingertip caresses.

Fun passion: She draws her initials on his chest.
Fervent passion: She leaves him speechless with her tender touch.

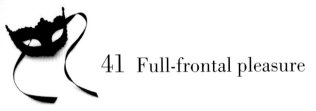

41 Full-frontal pleasure

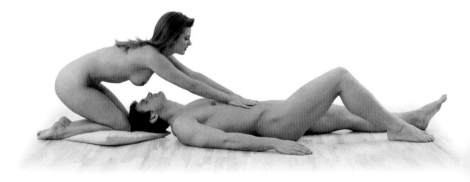

Tonight: She treats him to a massage that moves steadily south.

Quickie passion: Her oiled hands get her there in a second.
Lingering passion: She pauses for naughty nipple-to-nose caresses.

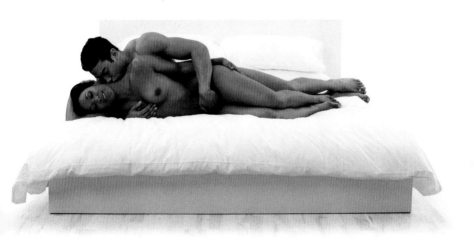

Tonight: He uses his hands to give her all-over-body shudders.

Quickie passion: He makes a fast and thrusting entrance from behind.
Lingering passion: He teases her with soft, slow circles of his fingers.

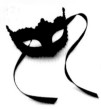

43 Rubbing him the right way

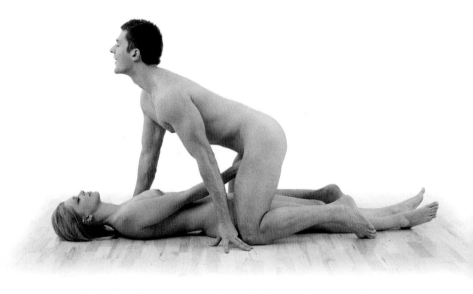

Tonight: She brings him joy with slick hand-over-hand strokes.

Beginner passion: She smoothes his shaft against his belly with oiled palms.
Sexpert passion: She slides down to give him a spit and polish.

Two-hand tango 44

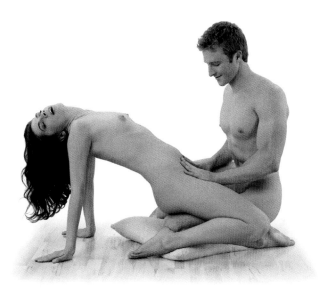

Tonight: He glides his fingers in fluid movements across her dance floor.

Quickie passion: She throws her head back, and thrusts her hips forward.
Lingering passion: He makes his moves slow slow, quick quick, slow.

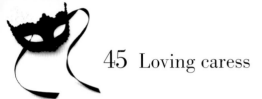

45 Loving caress

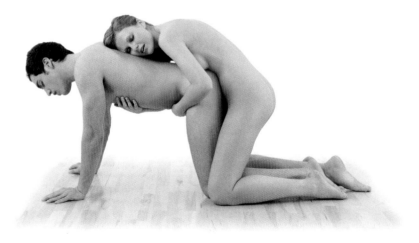

Tonight: She takes a sweet, loving approach to raising his manhood.

Fun passion: She tickles his balls and belly with her fingertips.
Fervent passion: She tells him with a moan how gorgeous he is.

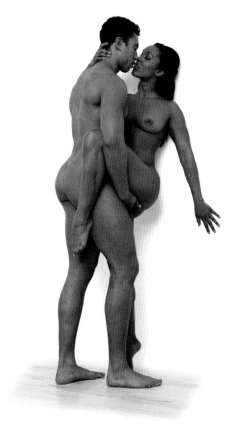

Tonight: He comes across all dominant, and gets naughty against a wall.

Beginner passion: He presses his lips to hers, and tickles her clitoris.
Sexpert passion: He lifts her up, and treats her to some joyous pump action.

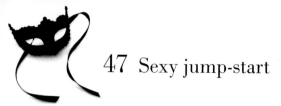

47 Sexy jump-start

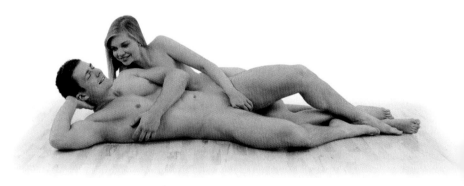

Tonight: She reaches around to charge his battery.

Clean passion: She caresses his back with her spare hand.
Kinky passion: She uses her spare hand to explore his butt.

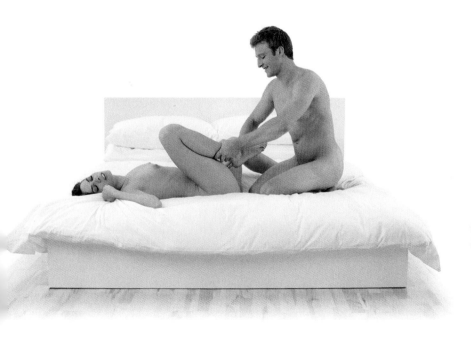

Tonight: He kneels at her feet, and smoothly opens her pleasure zone.

Sweet passion: He kisses her toes with soft lips.
Wild passion: She spreads her legs while he works with both hands.

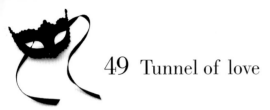

49 Tunnel of love

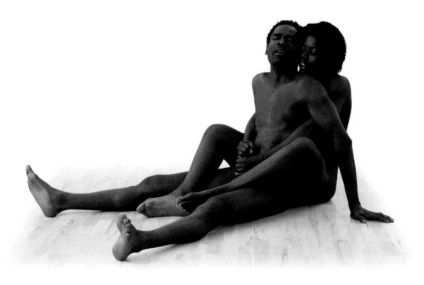

Tonight: She takes him for a smooth, slick ride in the tunnel of her hands.

Quickie passion: She pumps him without mercy.
Lingering passion: She pauses to fondle other local attractions.

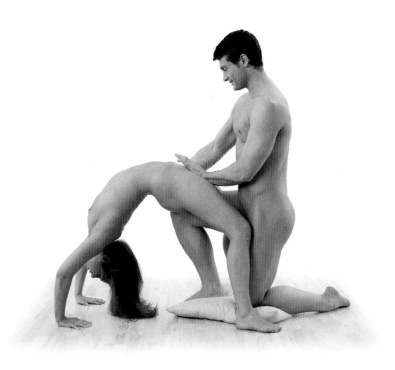

Tonight: He sends sweet sensations through her arched body.

Beginner passion: She comes down to come.
Sexpert passion: She stays up, and he catches her at the climax.

51 Prepared by hand

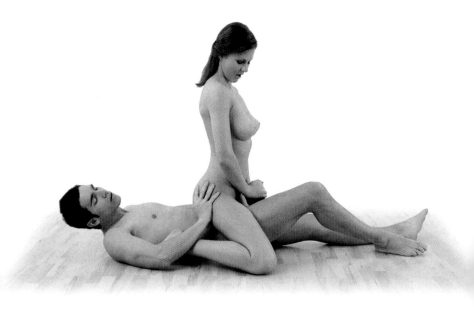

Tonight: She gets him ready for bed with both hands and a dollop of lube.

Clean passion: She shows him what a good sense of rhythm she's got.
Kinky passion: As he swells with desire she pops a penis ring on him.

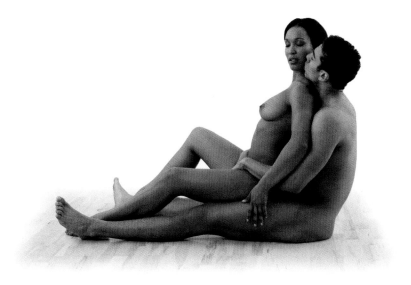

Tonight: He takes a leisurely approach to learning how to touch her.

Sweet passion: He caresses her love button and her belly at the same time.
Wild passion: He plunges his fingers inside her as he bites her neck.

53 Getting his ball rolling

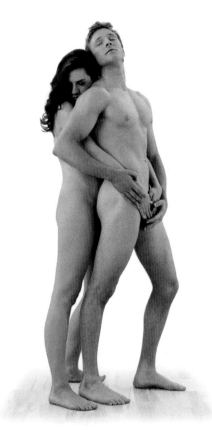

Tonight: She declares her intentions by curving her palms around his jewels.

Fun passion: She triggers a sudden growth spurt with her fingers.
Fervent passion: You sink to the ground together in blissful synchrony.

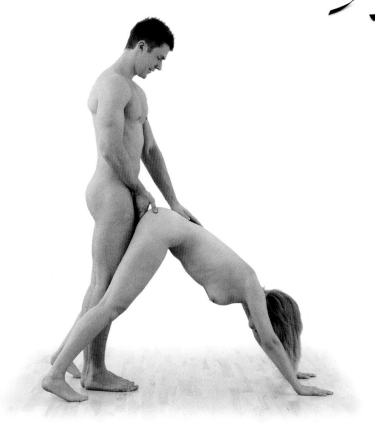

Tonight: He uses his hands sexily to disrupt her yoga practice.

Sweet passion: You end up cuddling on her yoga mat.
Wild passion: He throws his hard lingam into her downward dog.

55 Passionate prayer

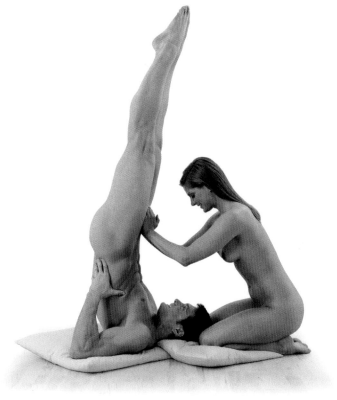

Tonight: She sets light to his candles as she kneels in prayer.

Quickie passion: She's done plenty of worshiping in advance.
Lingering passion: She turns it into a slow, sexy, Tantric meditation.

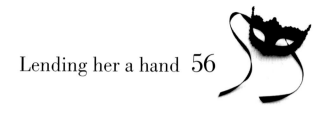

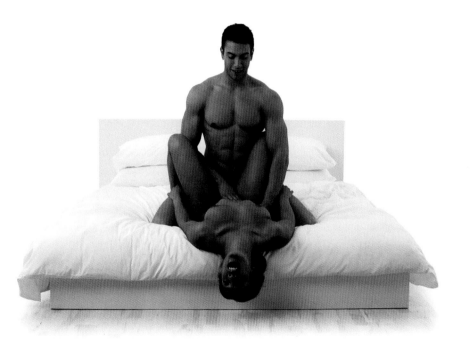

Tonight: He comes to her aid with an energetic hand.

Sweet passion: He asks her if he's doing it right.
Wild passion: He finishes the job by vibrating his tip hard against her.

57 Pleasure circuit

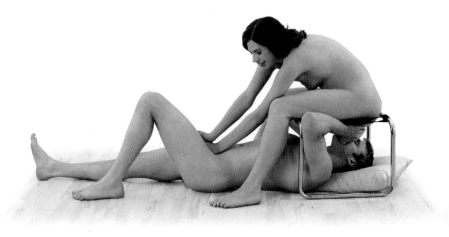

Tonight: He explores all the ways he can do her while she's doing him.

Fun passion: You see if it's possible while standing up.
Fervent passion: You time it so that you enter the O-zone together.

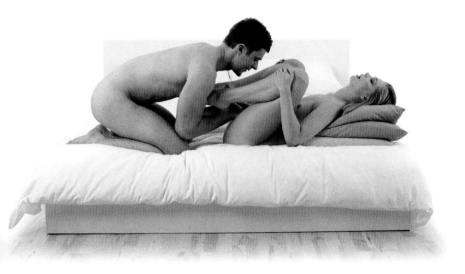

Tonight: He takes his fingers for a leisurely walk around her tulip garden.

Clean passion: He pauses to softly stroke her petals.
Kinky passion: He takes her to the edge by nipping her bud with his fingers.

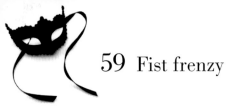

59 Fist frenzy

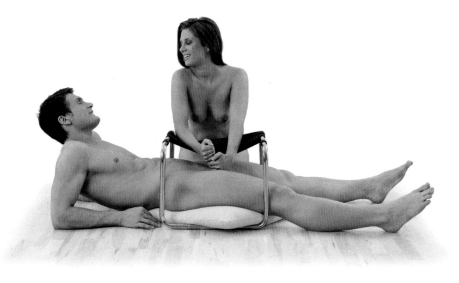

Tonight: She works him into a lather with her fists.

Quickie passion: He blissfully surrenders to the inevitable.
Lingering passion: She tugs his balls to bring him back from the peak.

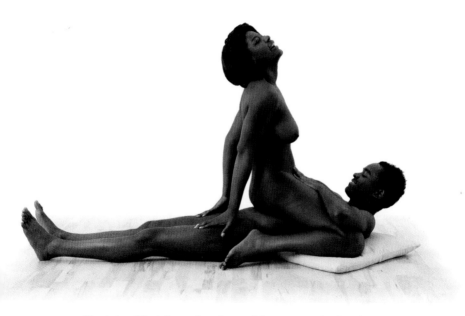

Tonight: He delivers her first red-hot orgasm by hand.

Beginner passion: She leans back, and lets him take charge.
Sexpert passion: She reaches behind, and takes him in hand too.

61 Naughty nurse

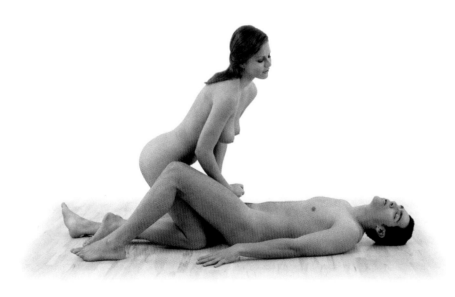

Tonight: He drifts into erotic heaven as she tenderly nurses his stiff bits.

Quickie passion: She takes a brisk, let's-get-the-job-done approach.
Lingering passion: She takes a leisurely, tickle-and-tease approach.

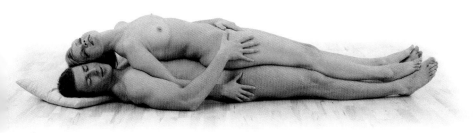

Tonight: She covers him while he blows her fuse with his fingers.

Clean passion: He finds a rhythm that makes her crackle.
Kinky passion: He makes her explode by talking dirty in her ear.

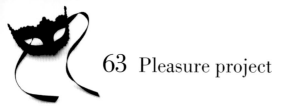

63 Pleasure project

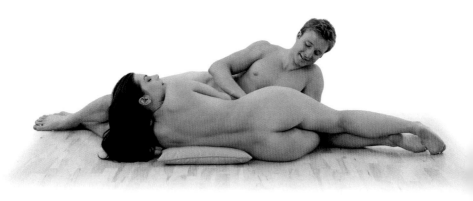

Tonight: You lie top to tail, then reach out and touch each other.

Quickie passion: You agree to work to a ferocious deadline.
Lingering passion: Your meeting meanders late into the night.

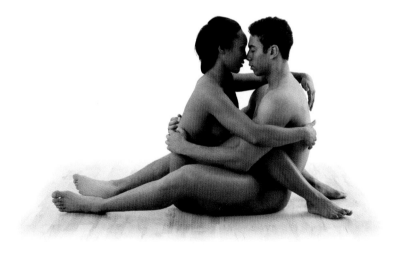

Tonight: You abandon yourselves to sex, strokes, cuddles, and fondles.

Beginner passion: You drizzle on oil, then draw swirls with your fingertips.
Sexpert passion: You go Tantric and breathe in erotic energy together.

65 The sweetest touch

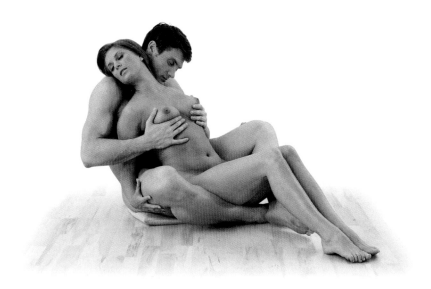

Tonight: He folds her into his arms for glorious mid-sex massages.

Clean passion: She relaxes into rapturous sensuality.
Kinky passion: He goes in super-hard on her nipples.

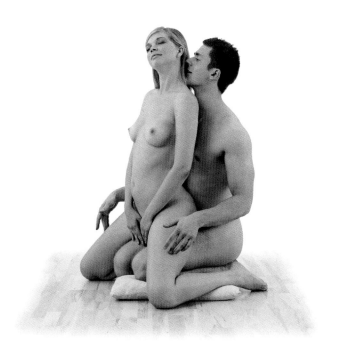

Tonight: He makes her shiver for hours with his feathery touch.

Fun passion: He wears gloves to give her a new sensation.
Fervent passion: He caresses her neck with his hot breath.

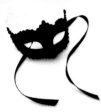

67 Mind-blowing backstroke

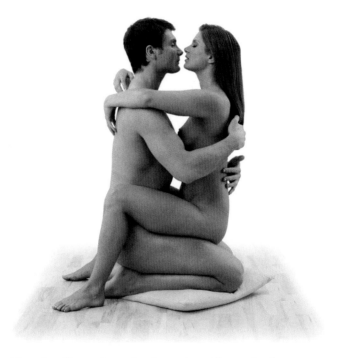

Tonight: You make each other swim with sexy back caresses.

Beginner passion: You add some breaststroke into the mix.
Sexpert passion: He pushes her back, and front crawls on top of her.

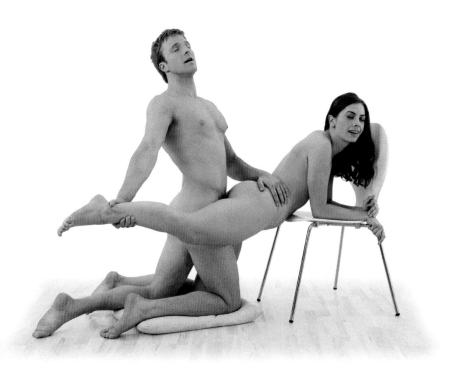

Tonight: He inserts his fifth limb, then offers her some movement therapy.

Fun passion: He pulls her playfully around the room.
Fervent passion: Her stretched-out limbs make him moan with delight.

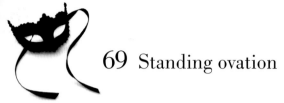

69 Standing ovation

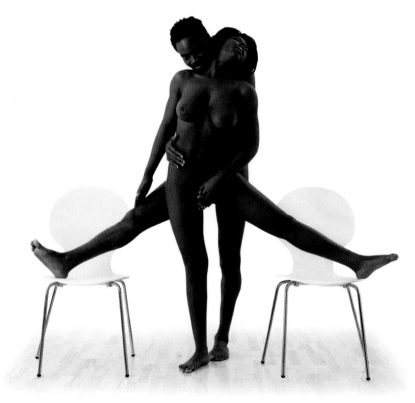

Tonight: He enters smoothly from behind, and applauds her with his hands.

Quickie passion: He moves so fast that there's time for an encore.
Lingering passion: He takes the slow, sensual route.

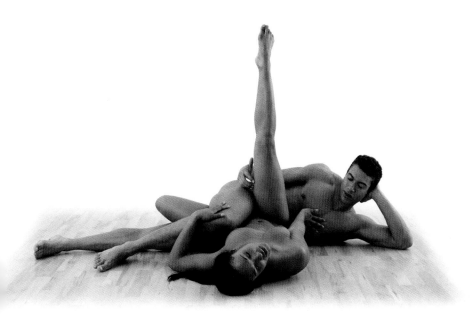

Tonight: She enjoys leg-in-the-air raunchiness while he fires the rocket fuel.

Quickie passion: He enters only when you're both at the 3-2-1 stage.
Lingering passion: You trail your fingers over each other, and go into orbit.

71 Sensual straddle

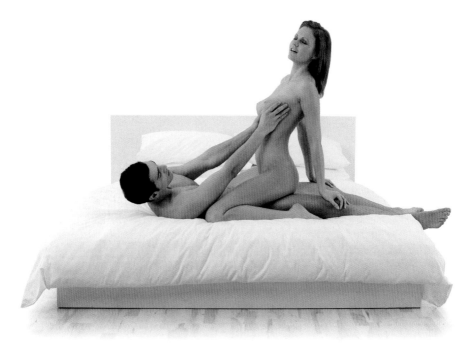

Tonight: She starts out as she means to go on—on top.

Clean passion: He leans forward, and cups her breasts in his hands.
Kinky passion: He sits up, and naughtily wraps her twins around his face.

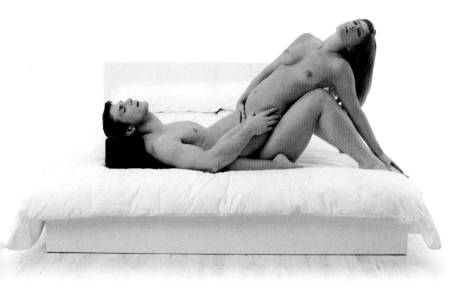

Tonight: She climbs on top the moment that she gets in from work.

Beginner passion: He strokes her body to get her hot.
Sexpert passion: He's pre-prepared her by sending her dirty texts all day.

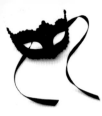

73 Yearning curve

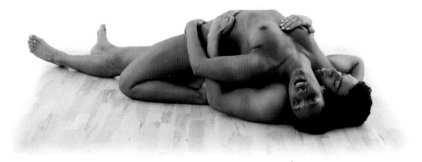

Tonight: You revel in stretched-out sensations that ripple through you both.

Sweet passion: He caresses her curves with his hot hands.
Wild passion: She drives him into a frenzy of desire with her gyrations.

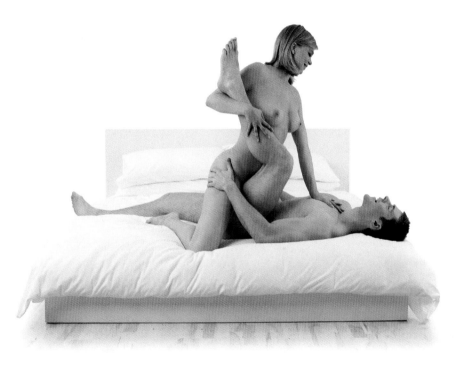

Tonight: She makes it her job to bend, stretch, and pull until she's satisfied.

Clean passion: She treats it as though it's an evening of exercise.
Kinky passion: She gets a naughty thrill from pushing his pain boundaries.

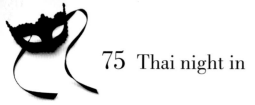

75 Thai night in

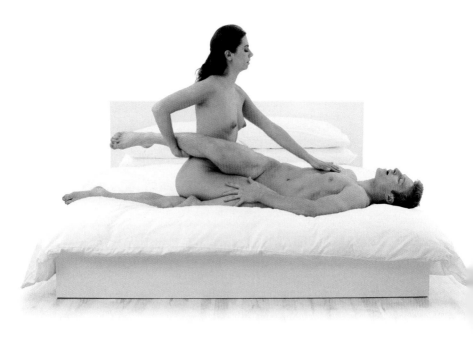

Tonight: You stay at home for some Thai-style massage.

Sweet passion: She promises him a happy ending.
Wild passion: She feverishly rubs his jade stalk with her oiled hands.

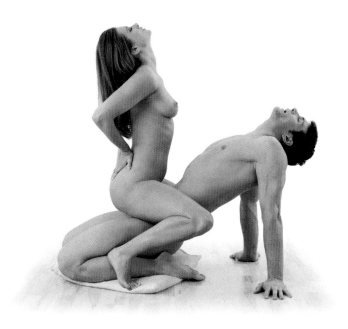

Tonight: He offers his body to her to slip and slide on.

Quickie passion: She slithers like a wild woman.
Lingering passion: She keeps her hair on.

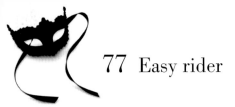

77 Easy rider

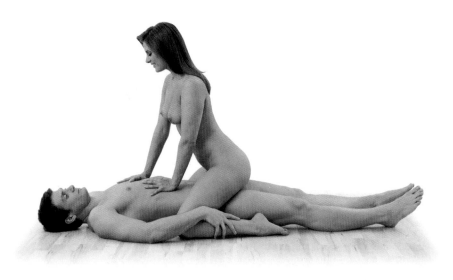

Tonight: She takes the reins in a range of sure-thing positions.

Clean passion: She gazes lovingly at him.
Kinky passion: She talks filthy while she rides.

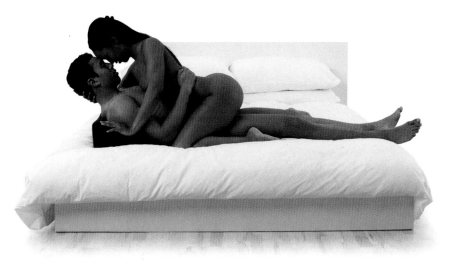

Tonight: She asks him to lie back, so that she can make the moves.

Fun passion: She plays the man; he plays the woman.
Fervent passion: She tells him in a breathy whisper how good he feels inside.

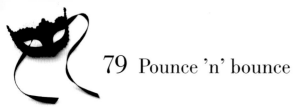

79 Pounce 'n' bounce

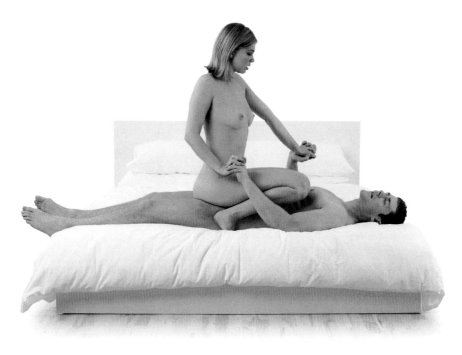

Tonight: She treats him to a selection of her best bouncy positions.

Beginner passion: She soothes him with slow mini-bounces.
Sexpert passion: She makes his eyes water with fast up-and-down pounding.

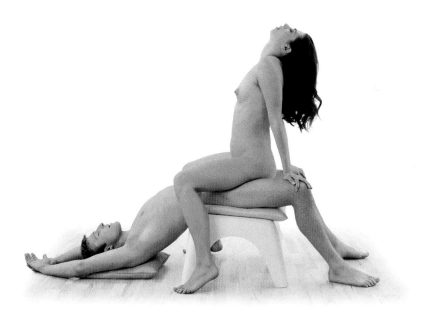

Tonight: She rides on top of his high wave.

Fun passion: She wears a fetish-style wetsuit.
Fervent passion: She moans with euphoria as she feels him surge.

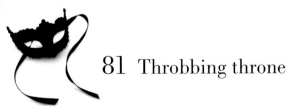

81 Throbbing throne

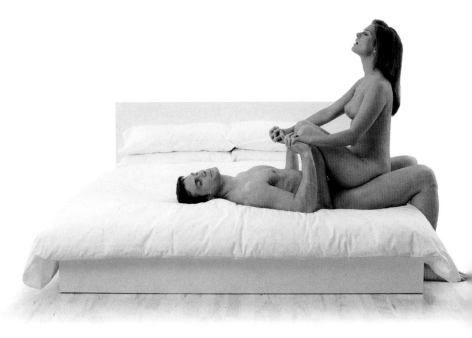

Tonight: She assumes her rightful regal position for the evening.

Sweet passion: He plays the role of her solid underling.
Wild passion: He overthrows her monarchy, and leaps on top.

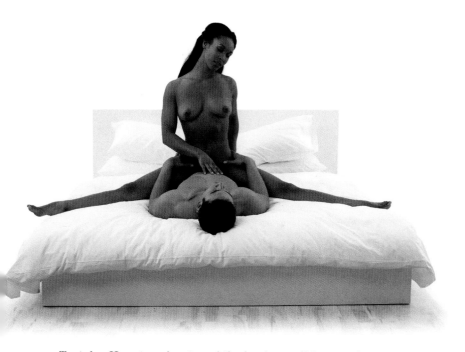

Tonight: He enjoys the view while she shows off her suppleness.

Fun passion: She ups the titillation with some naughty nipple tassels.
Fervent passion: You gaze into each other's eyes as the tension mounts.

83 Ripple 'n' slink

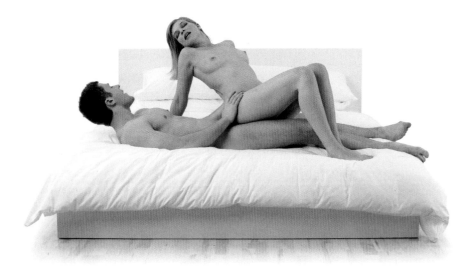

Tonight: She sensually slinks on top of him for some smooth undulations.

Quickie passion: She does it after giving him a body-rocking blowjob.
Lingering passion: She puts on some slow, slinky music.

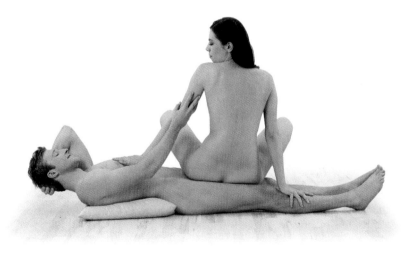

Tonight: She sits down on him when he's not expecting it.

Beginner passion: She coaxes him with caresses.
Sexpert passion: She gets under his skin by talking dirty.

85 Warming his bench

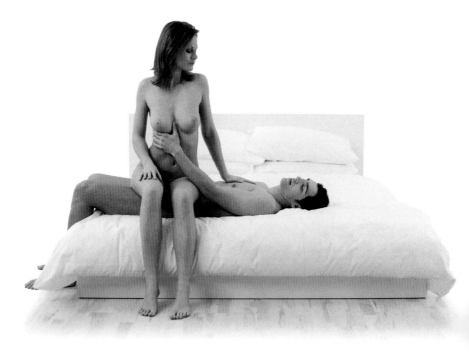

Tonight: You pretend to be sexy strangers meeting in the park.

Fun passion: She acts innocent and claims she just wants a seat.
Fervent passion: You both succumb to an unstoppable kissing session.

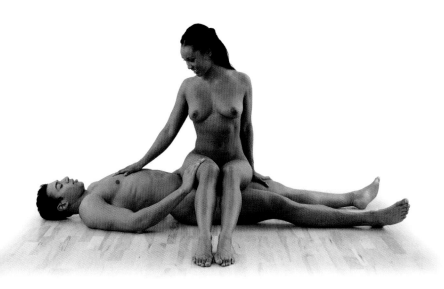

Tonight: You dedicate the evening to side-entry sex.

Clean passion: She whets his appetite with her little waist wiggles.
Kinky passion: She dresses as a nun, and pretends it's her first time.

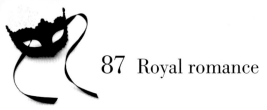

87 Royal romance

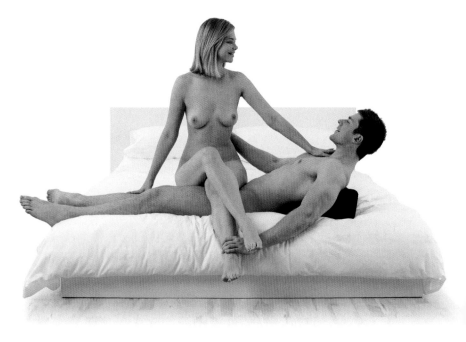

Tonight: She plays the horny queen to his lusty king.

Fun passion: You address each other as "Your majesty".
Fervent passion: She convulses with pleasure as his scepter enters her.

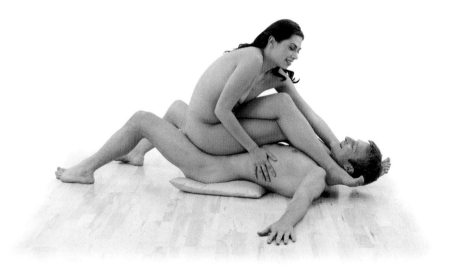

Tonight: She feels the joy of keeping her legs crossed.

Beginner passion: She leaves a handy gap for her fingers.
Sexpert passion: She builds up frenetic friction between them.

89 Shake, straddle, and roll

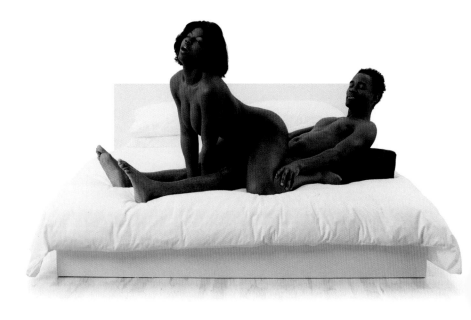

Tonight: She drives him crazy with loose talk and fast moves.

Fun passion: She cheekily shakes her butt while glancing back at him.
Fervent passion: He gives in to whole-body trembles of lust.

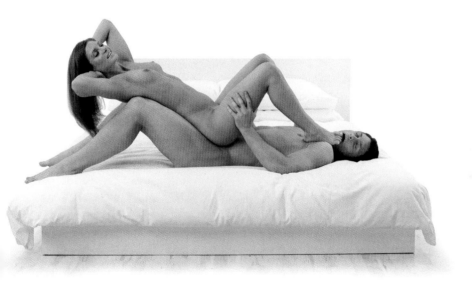

Tonight: She lies back, and suns herself on his beach.

Sweet passion: She reaches down to fondle his rocks.
Wild passion: He takes her for an exciting ride on the crest of his wave.

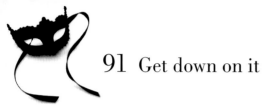

91 Get down on it

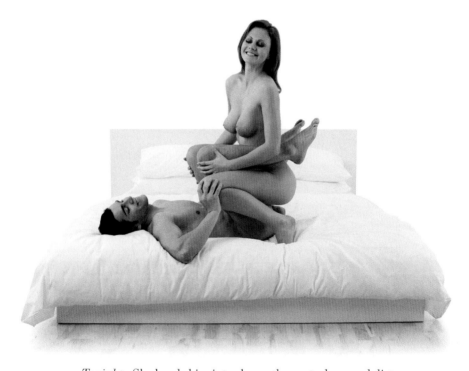

Tonight: She bends him into shape, then gets down and dirty.

Clean passion: She grabs his knees, and gives the mattress a pounding.
Kinky passion: She gives him a smile, and pops on a collar and leash.

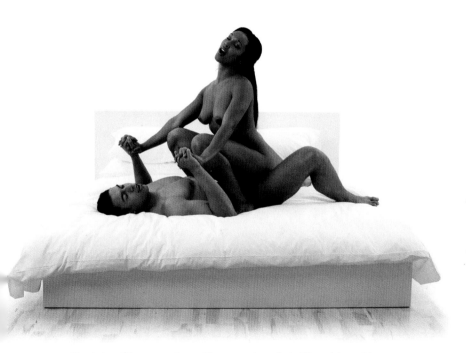

Tonight: She treats herself to a series of thrill-seeking rides.

Quickie passion: She bumps and grinds to a barely containable big "O".
Lingering passion: She massages his pole with slow, up-and-down strokes.

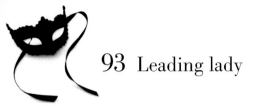

93 Leading lady

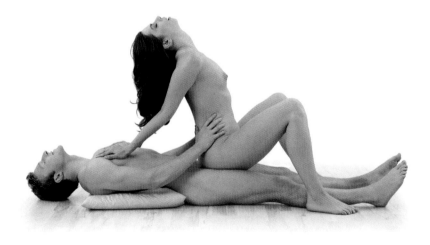

Tonight: She brings him an evening of taut sexual tension and drama.

Fun passion: She won't perform until the cameras roll.
Fervent passion: She throws her head back, and moans his name.

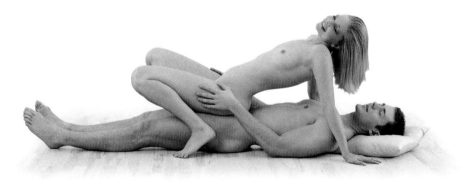

Tonight: She explores the angles that give her maximum thrust.

Sweet passion: He adds a friendly hand to assist her rhythm.
Wild passion: He grabs her, and spins her over into doggie position.

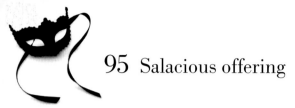

95 Salacious offering

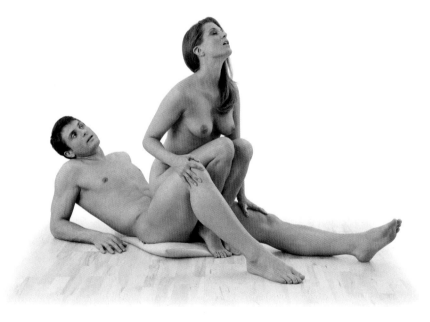

Tonight: He offers her a firm and comfortable seat for the night.

Fun passion: She agrees to try him out for size.
Fervent passion: She's instantly at his erotic mercy.

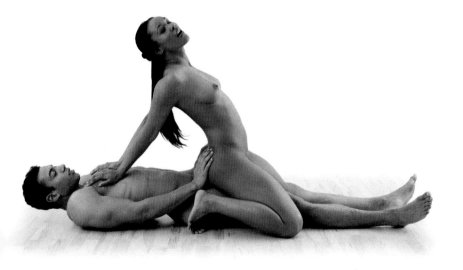

Tonight: You relish anonymity in a saucy line-up of rear-entry positions.

Clean passion: You fantasize about the best sex you've had with your partner.
Kinky passion: You fantasize about having sex with your favorite celebrity.

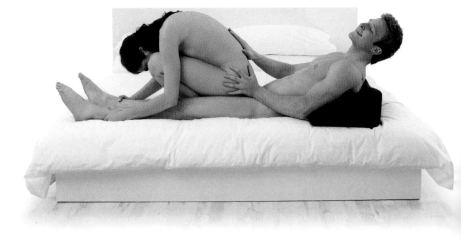

Tonight: He takes her out of this world with a sex-plus-backrub session.

Beginner passion: He keeps his probe still while massaging her.
Sexpert passion: He moves everything at once to give her a cosmic climax.

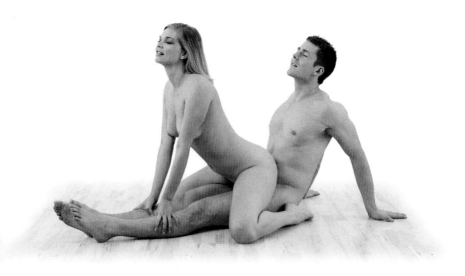

Tonight: She straddles him cowgirl-style, and figures out the best angles.

Fun passion: She wears a cowgirl hat, and chews a blade of grass.
Fervent passion: He moans as he watches her sliding on and off.

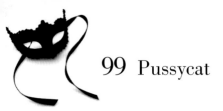

99 Pussycat

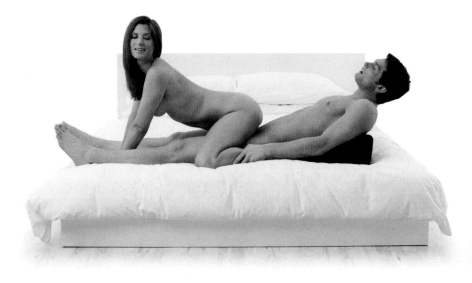

Tonight: She slinks on top, and becomes his adorable sex kitten.

Sweet passion: She covers him in tiny cat licks.
Wild passion: She bites and claws her way to a mewling climax.

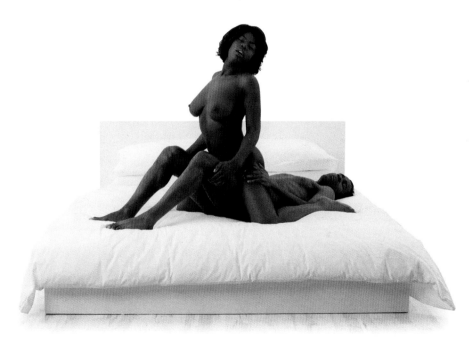

Tonight: She teasingly turns her back, and helps herself to him.

Clean passion: He lifts his head up so that he can see her.
Kinky passion: He gives her an X-rated commentary as he watches.

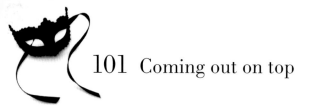

101 Coming out on top

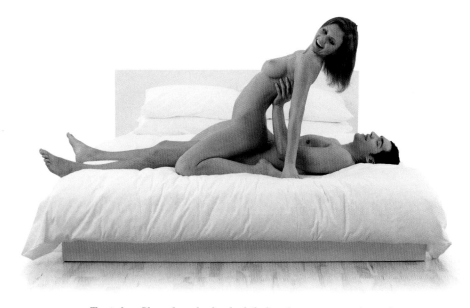

Tonight: She takes the lead while he plays a supporting role.

Quickie passion: She moves as if she's on a bucking bronco.
Lingering passion: He makes her shiver with light caresses along her spine.

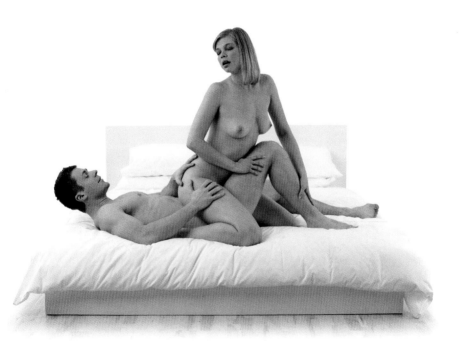

Tonight: She sets the night on fire by snaking herself around his thigh.

Clean passion: She slithers gently up and down.
Kinky passion: He offers to pop his python in her back door.

103 Glorious grinding

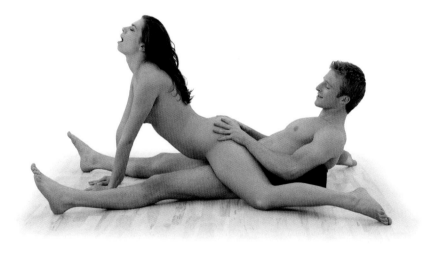

Tonight: She glides and grinds her way to paradise.

Sweet passion: She teases him by brushing his knees with her nipples.
Wild passion: She treats him to rapid missionary-style thrusts.

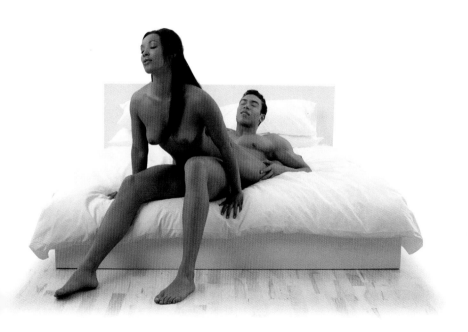

Tonight: She plays like a woman at the top of her game.

Quickie passion: She aims to hit the high notes first time.
Lingering passion: She builds slowly to an overwhelming crescendo.

105 Keeping him in tow

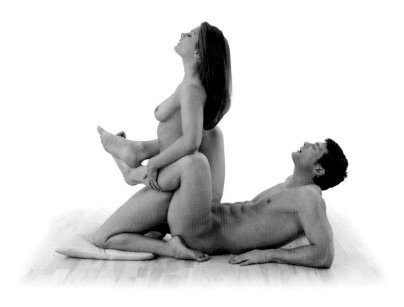

Tonight: She hitches up, and keeps him close behind all night.

Beginner passion: She carries his load carefully.
Sexpert passion: She pulls him so hard that he bounces off the walls.

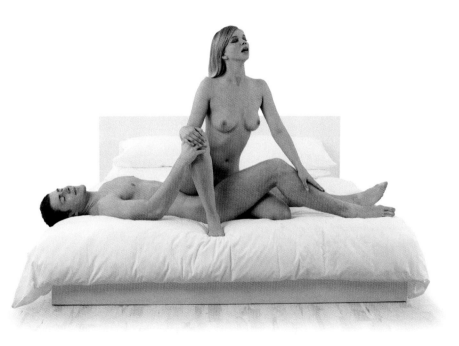

Tonight: After much teasing, she honors his love lord by slipping on top.

Quickie passion: She goes to work at a frenetic pace.
Lingering passion: She sits back on her heels when things overheat.

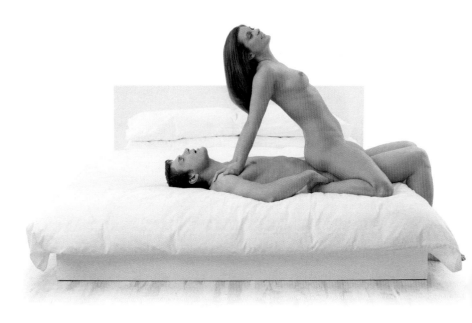

107 Private assistant

Tonight: He gives her some personally tailored back-up.

Clean passion: He asks her if there's anything that she'd like to delegate.
Kinky passion: He quivers with slavish devotion.

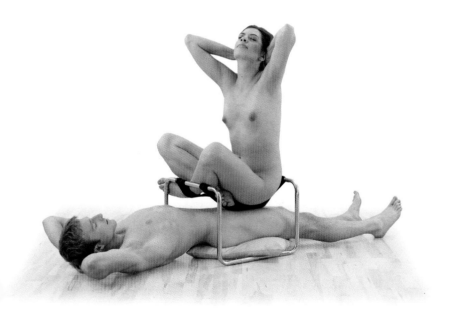

Tonight: She hovers on top as he visits her moon.

Beginner passion: He frolics in her outer orbit.
Sexpert passion: His hard entry sets off a moonquake.

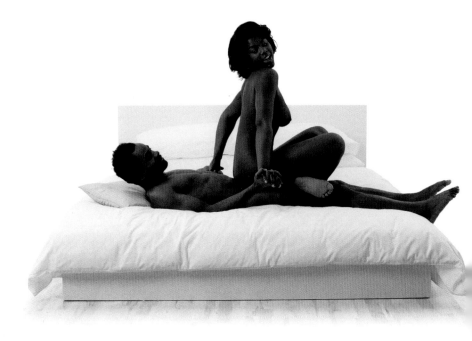

Tonight: She finds the sexiest ways to use up all his column space.

Sweet passion: She holds him lovingly tight from inside.
Wild passion: Her slipping, sliding moves rob him of all self-control.

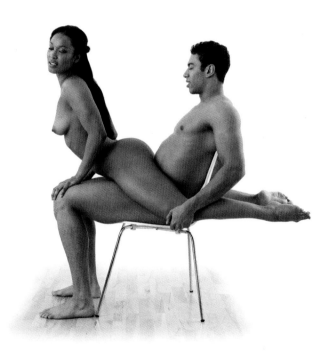

Tonight: She basks radiantly on his lap while he sits back and admires her.

Fun passion: Her ass cheeks read "Stroke me".
Fervent passion: You grind against each other to get the tightest possible fit.

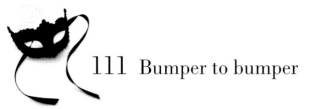

111 Bumper to bumper

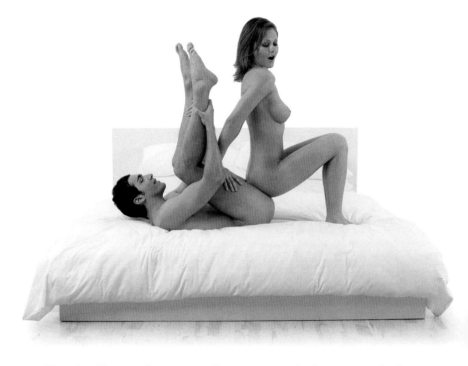

Tonight: She gets the evening off to a racy start by bouncing on his bumper.

Beginner passion: She obeys a slow speed limit.
Sexpert passion: She oils his spark plug to make things extra slippery.

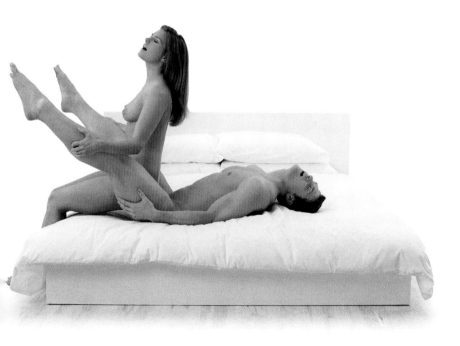

Tonight: She's in the driver's seat, and he's up for some firm steering.

Sweet passion: She compliments him on his gear shift.
Wild passion: Her driving is rampant and reckless.

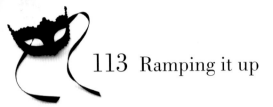

113 Ramping it up

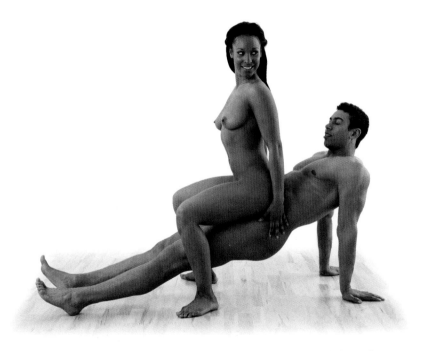

Tonight: He uses his body like a sex ramp for her slippery, sliding pleasure.

Clean passion: She climbs on board, and bounces her way to bliss.
Kinky passion: She punishes him if his butt touches the ground.

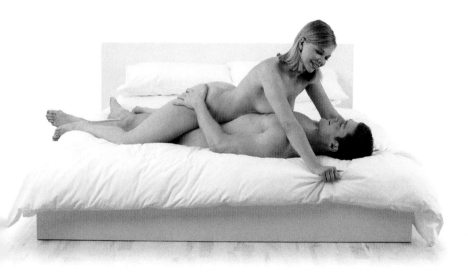

Tonight: She gives into her lust in a series of vigorous sheet-ripping moves.

Quickie passion: She finds the fast grind that makes her happy.
Lingering passion: He strokes her back to calm her ardor.

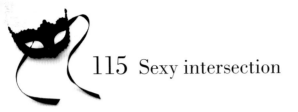

115 Sexy intersection

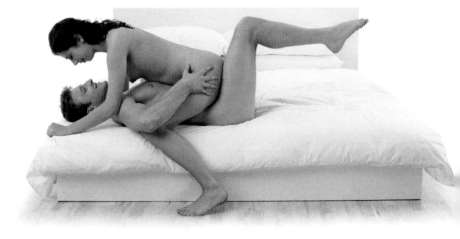

Tonight: He lies back while she forms a series of juicy junctions.

Fun passion: She begs him to enter her slippery road.
Fervent passion: You clasp each other tight, and go with the flow.

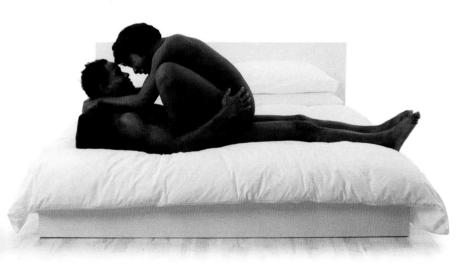

Tonight: She takes him in, and inflames him with erotic stories.

Quickie passion: She makes the plots depraved and debauched.
Lingering passion: She makes the plots sensual and seductive.

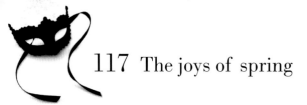

117 The joys of spring

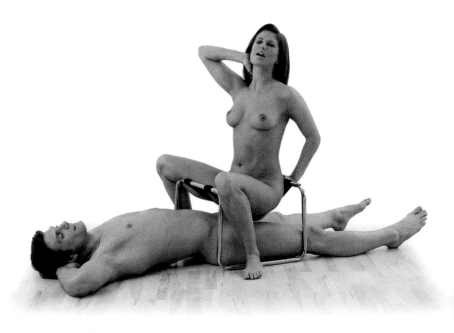

Tonight: He lies back while she springs the night away.

Sweet passion: He enhances her bounce power by cupping her cheeks.
Wild passion: She grabs the chair, and rocks her way to summer.

Back-to-front bounce 118

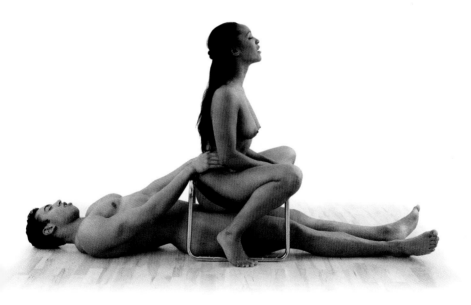

Tonight: She turns her back, and you both enter fantasy world.

Beginner passion: You share your sweet and sensual thoughts.
Sexpert passion: You share your dark and kinky thoughts.

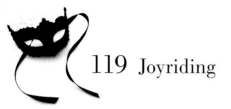

119 Joyriding

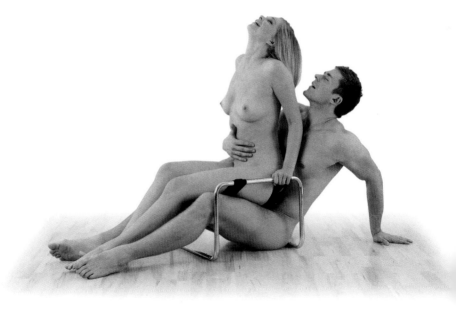

Tonight: She chooses to go on an erotic rampage.

Fun passion: He lets her smash and grab him.
Fervent passion: He echoes her shouts of joy.

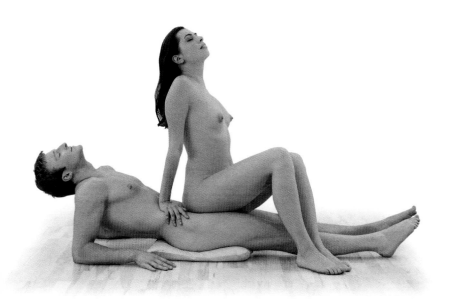

Tonight: She slides on top, and milks him with her muscles.

Sweet passion: She wears a short cotton dress.
Wild passion: She milks him with her mouth too.

121 Coming equipped for the job

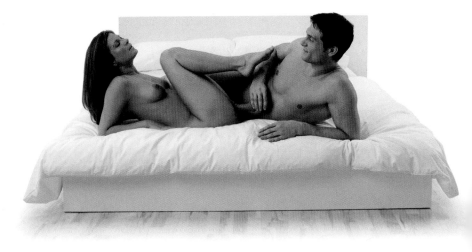

Tonight: He treats her to a buzzing and thrusting session.

Clean passion: He warms her up with a back massage.
Kinky passion: He leaves no opening unbuzzed.

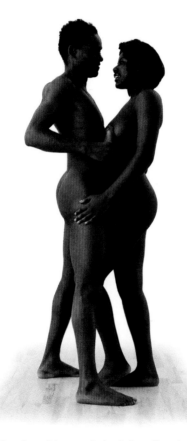

Tonight: He makes her shiver and tingle by vibrating her peak places.

Quickie passion: She pushes the vibrator right to where she wants it.
Lingering passion: He buzzes her top bits, and descends in his own time.

123 Saucy power surge

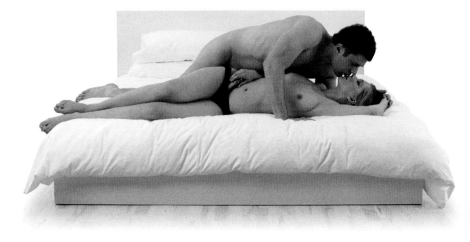

Tonight: You share a turbo-charged snog—she's got a vibrator in her pants.

Quickie passion: He jumps on top, and adds his own power supply.
Lingering passion: She turns the vibrator to a discreetly low purr.

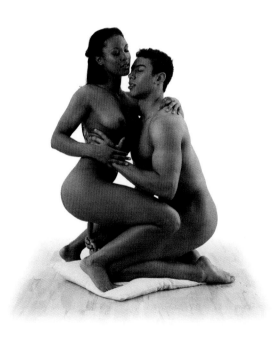

Tonight: He holds a vibrator firmly in his hand, and she takes it in slowly.

Beginner passion: She finds bliss by bobbing up and down on the tip.
Sexpert passion: He targets her G-spot, then flicks the vibe speed to max.

125 Hot vibrations

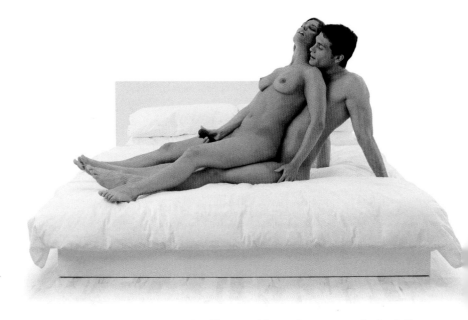

Tonight: He provides the filling, and leaves her to provide the frills.

Fun passion: He places a pile of batteries beside the bed.
Fervent passion: He holds her tight as she has one climax after another.

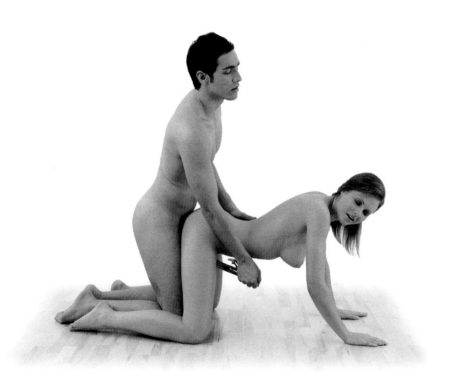

Tonight: You try the perfect pair: a rampant rabbit plus the doggie position.

Sweet passion: He makes her twitch before he does.
Wild passion: You both yelp with uncontrollable lust.

127 Giving him a fast buck

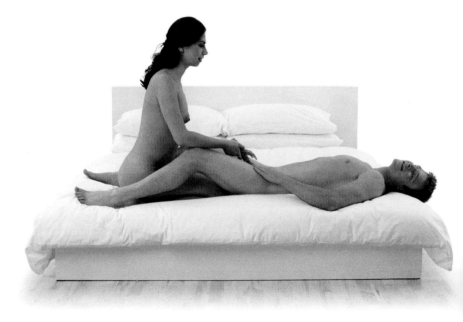

Tonight: She proves that men love rabbit sessions too.

Beginner passion: She vibrates the F-spot on his end.
Sexpert passion: She plunges inside to vibrate his P-spot.

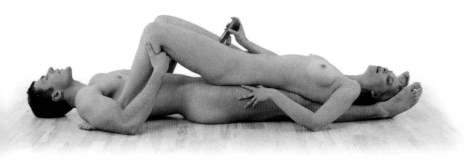

Tonight: You lie back and lose yourself in fantasy—and sexy vibrations.

Sweet passion: She shares the vibes between the two of you.
Wild passion: You describe your fantasies to each other in dirty detail.

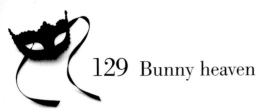

129 Bunny heaven

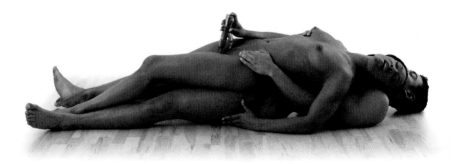

Tonight: She settles into joyous vibrations delivered to her front and back.

Quickie passion: She targets her hot spot with the rabbit ears.
Lingering passion: She hops the rabbit from her to him, then back again.

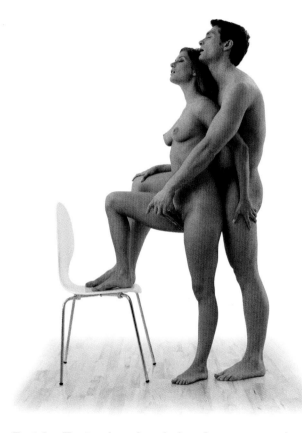

Tonight: He gives her a buzz before she goes out on the town.

Fun passion: She smiles and winks as she walks out the door.
Fervent passion: She misses him, and comes home within the hour.

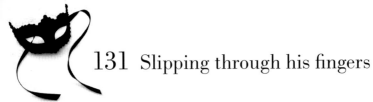

131 Slipping through his fingers

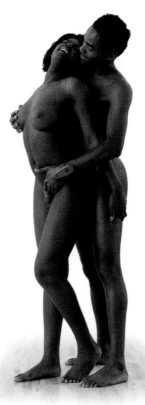

Tonight: He brings her joy with a vibrating hand that never tires.

Beginner passion: He services her standing up.
Sexpert passion: He services her standing, sitting, and upside-down.

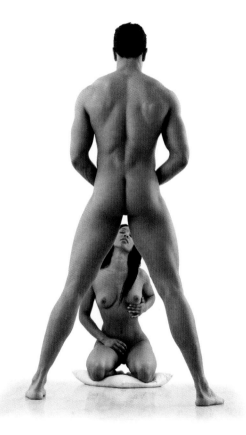

Tonight: You watch each other indulge in some manual self-love.

Quickie passion: You compete vigorously to reach the finish line.
Lingering passion: You repeatedly pull back from the brink of ecstasy.

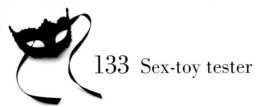

133 Sex-toy tester

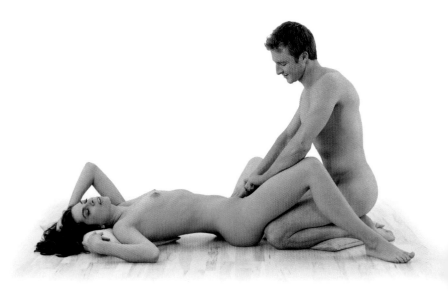

Tonight: He investigates which sex toys press her buttons.

Clean passion: She awards each toy a star rating.
Kinky passion: He joins her to test a double dildo.

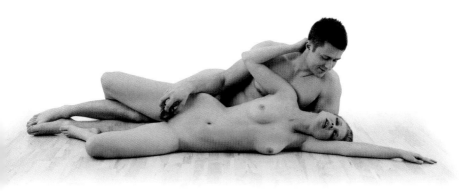

Tonight: He makes her moist and breathless with a handy pebble vibrator.

Beginner passion: He gives all his attention to her front.
Sexpert passion: He inserts something filling from behind at the same time.

135 Sex that goes buzz in the night

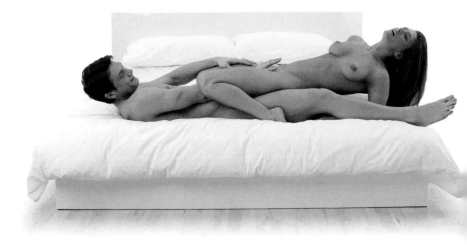

Tonight: He surprises her with a buzzer in the palm of his hand.

Quickie passion: He drives her wild with maximum vibrations.
Lingering passion: He goes for a slow burn.

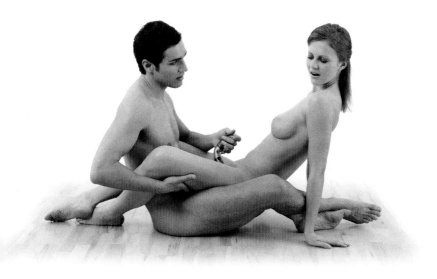

Tonight: He targets her G-spot with the aid of a bendy vibrator.

Sweet passion: He gives her a melting erotic massage beforehand.
Wild passion: He uses the vibrator to give her a body-writhing orgasm.

137 Rear admiral

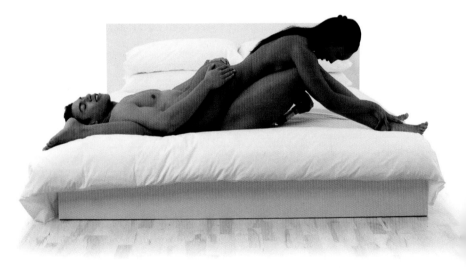

Tonight: You make forays into each other's forbidden territories.

Beginner passion: You agree which lines you can or can't cross.
Sexpert passion: He rewards her hot vibrations with tingling spanks.

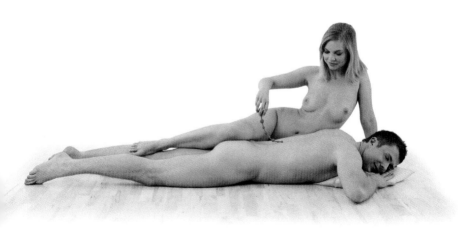

Tonight: She makes him close his eyes, and guess the sex toy of the night.

Sweet passion: She gives him another guess when he gets it wrong.
Wild passion: She brazenly inserts the toy into him if he gets it wrong.

139 Decorating her with beads

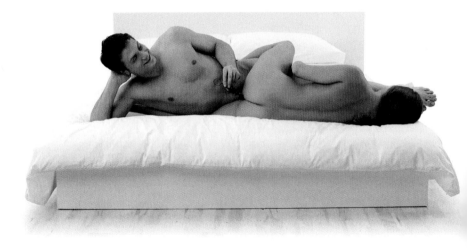

Tonight: He tries out some beady back-door experiments.

Fun passion: She bites if it gets too much.
Fervent passion: He uses his own tool to make a throbbing entry.

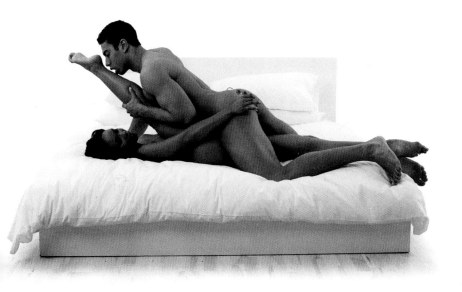

Tonight: He presses himself into her as she presses anal beads into him.

Clean passion: She starts with some innocent buttock caresses.
Kinky passion: He offers to decorate her with a pearl necklace.

141 Double whammy

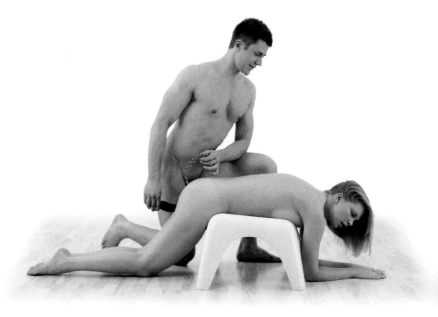

Tonight: He makes her legs tremble by using two sex toys at the same time.

Beginner passion: He doesn't try to do too much at once.
Sexpert passion: He's a fast and raunchy multitasker.

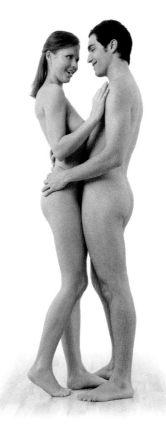

Tonight: She reveals her secret tool for turbo-charged blowjobs.

Fun passion: She slips a vibrator on his tongue too, and suggests a 69.
Fervent passion: She falls to her knees because she wants him so badly.

143 Saucy shopper

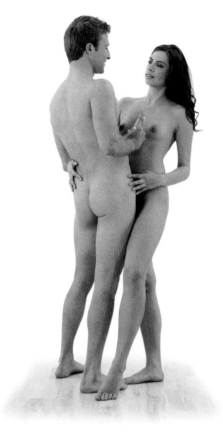

Tonight: He reveals the naughty purchase that he's just made.

Quickie passion: He throws her on the bed, and gives the toy a test drive.
Lingering passion: He describes his plans for her in lavish detail first.

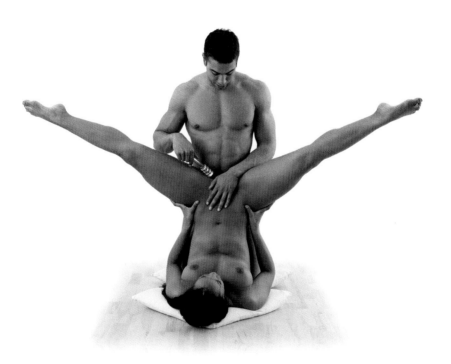

Tonight: She opens herself up to the velvety touch of a glass dildo.

Sweet passion: He warms it first, then rotates it gently inside her.
Wild passion: He slips it into her shallow end, then bobs it in and out.

145 Lip fantastic

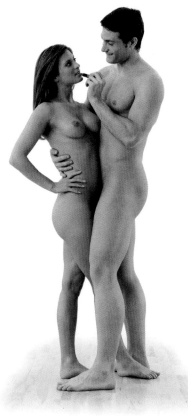

Tonight: He uses a lipstick vibrator to make her feel gorgeous.

Beginner passion: He kisses the tingles away afterward.
Sexpert passion: He "paints" both sets of lips.

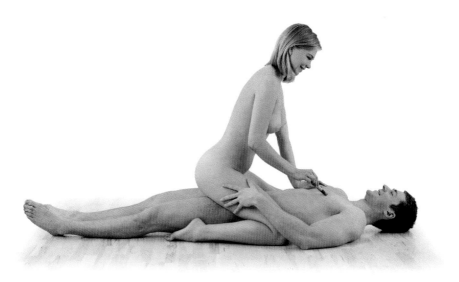

Tonight: She uses a tiny vibrator to map out new erogenous zones.

Clean passion: She stays firmly in his upper territories.
Kinky passion: She dives straight into his undergrowth.

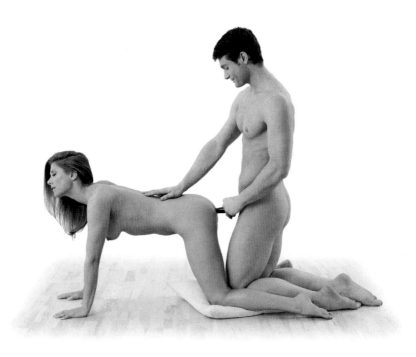

Tonight: He uses a vibrating butt plug to stretch her boundaries.

Beginner passion: He breaks her in with a lubed finger.
Sexpert passion: He strokes her clit too, and gives her sensational spasms.

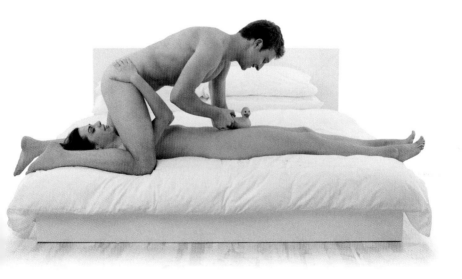

Tonight: You make each other smile with a ducking and diving session.

Sweet passion: He has a turn on the duck too.
Wild passion: You try the thrashy, splashy bath version.

149 Dirty duck

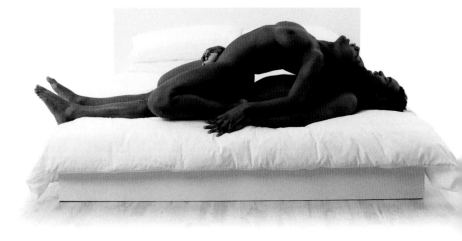

Tonight: She brings a friend to bed—her duck vibrator.

Quickie passion: She pushes the duck between her legs, and thrusts hard.
Lingering passion: She and the duck move in sensual harmony.

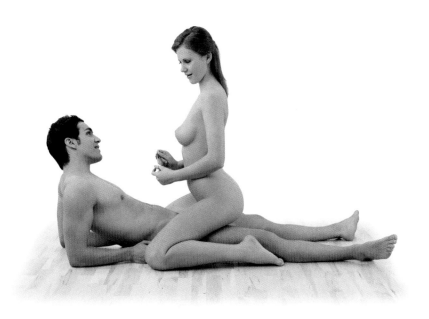

Tonight: She presents him with a penis ring, and vows to ride him hard.

Fun passion: She makes him promise to love, honor, and obey her in bed.
Fervent passion: She moans ecstatically as she slips the ring over his shaft.

151 Filling her with love

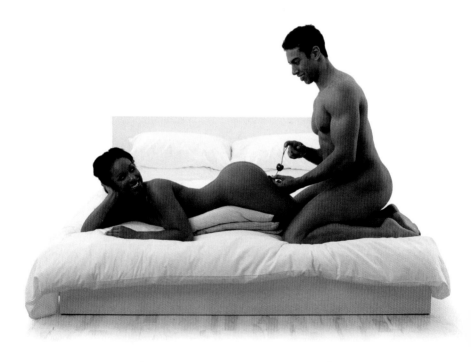

Tonight: She lies on her front to receive his gift of love balls.

Sweet passion: He leans forward to nuzzle and lick her cleft.
Wild passion: He slides his manhood in and out between her mounds.

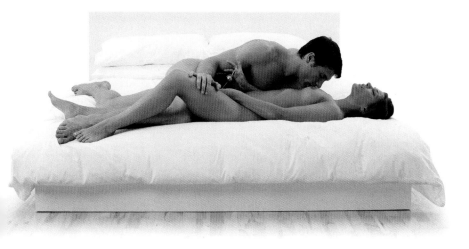

Tonight: She reveals that she's been wearing love balls all day…

Clean passion: He jumps on top to soak up her lust.
Kinky passion: He reveals that he's been wearing nipple clamps all day.

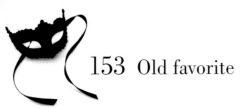

153 Old favorite

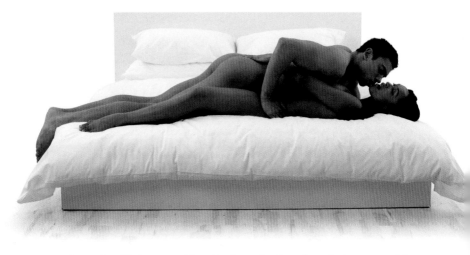

Tonight: He begins with a timeless classic—the missionary position.

Quickie passion: He moves his hips with the speed of a jackhammer.
Lingering passion: He takes breaks to slide down and tongue her treasures.

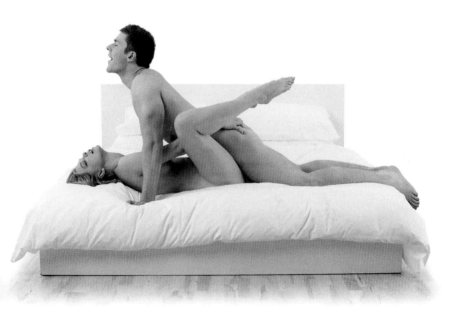

Tonight: She welcomes him home with a series of come-on-in positions.

Sweet passion: She's waiting in bed for him.
Wild passion: She grabs his buttocks, and rams him into her.

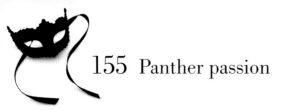

155 Panther passion

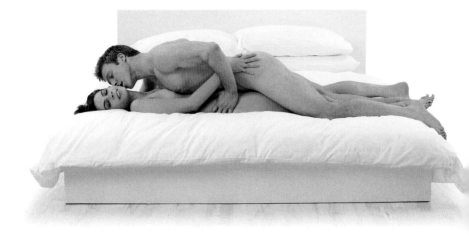

Tonight: He slinks up her body while she's sleeping.

Fun passion: He says: "Do you want to come in my cougar?"
Fervent passion: He shows his teeth and growls ravenously.

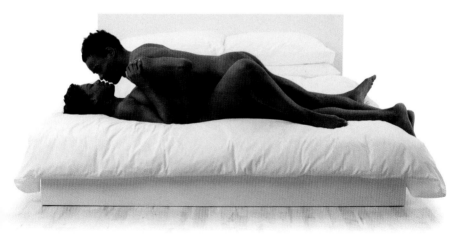

Tonight: You devote yourselves to missionary-inspired positions.

Fun passion: She says: "Do you come here often?"
Fervent passion: You spend the night kissing and nuzzling each other.

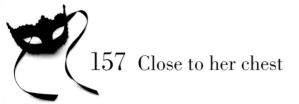

157 Close to her chest

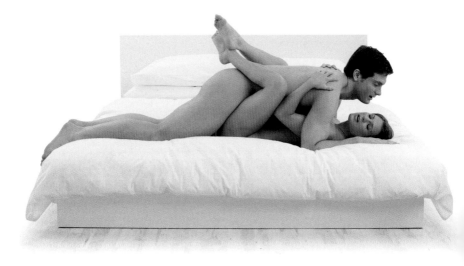

Tonight: He gets carnally close, and stays there.

Beginner passion: You work up some intense genital friction.
Sexpert passion: You share a whole-body, Tantric orgasm.

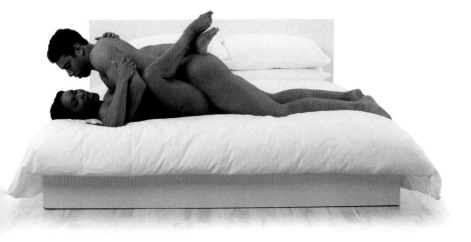

Tonight: Try some hot positions in which she sets the pace with her feet.

Clean passion: She pulls him in tight, and you both savor the moment.
Kinky passion: She does it while wearing her highest, spikiest stilettos.

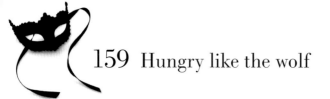

159 Hungry like the wolf

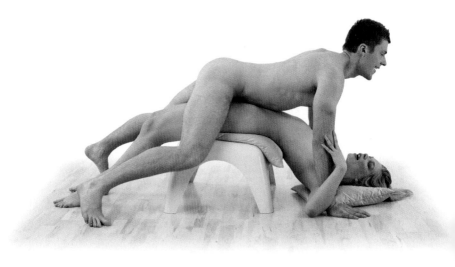

Tonight: He shows her exactly how big his appetite is.

Sweet passion: He promises to be gentle.
Wild passion: He takes breaks to snap his tongue between her legs.

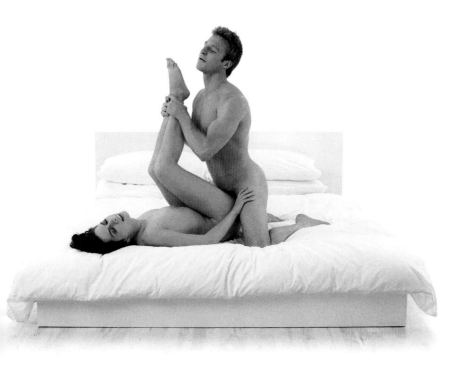

Tonight: He shows his devotional side in an evening of reverent sex.

Quickie passion: She blasphemes, and pushes him over the edge.
Lingering passion: He closes his eyes, and kisses her sole.

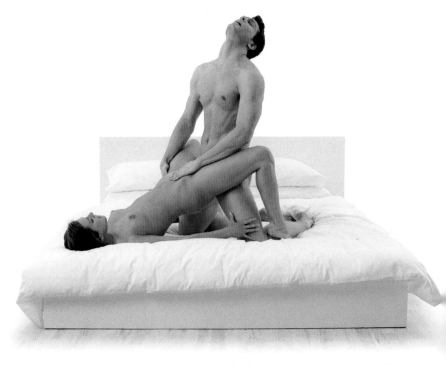

Tonight: He kneels squarely on the bed, and she rises to the occasion.

Beginner passion: She stays still, and he thrusts.
Sexpert passion: She does her best belly-dancing moves.

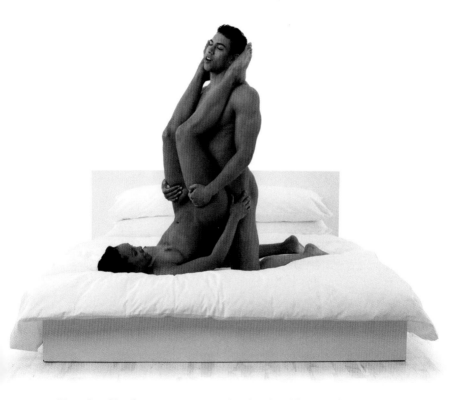

Tonight: She demonstrates exactly why shoulder-stands are sexy.

Fun passion: He positions himself opposite to a full-length mirror.
Fervent passion: He slides into her slowly after an hour of intense foreplay.

163 Yearning yogi

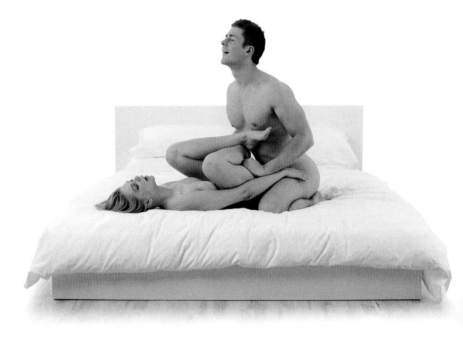

Tonight: She bends herself into erotic yoga positions, and he climbs on top.

Clean passion: You pant in time with each other.
Kinky passion: He holds her ankles tightly so that there's no escape.

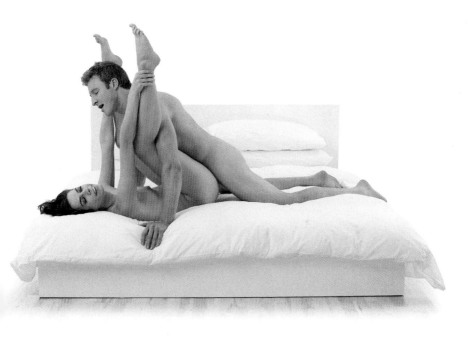

Tonight: You have no-holds-barred porn-star-style sex into the early hours.

Beginner passion: You throw yourselves joyously into multiple positions.
Sexpert passion: You climax together ecstatically on cue.

165 Lap of lust

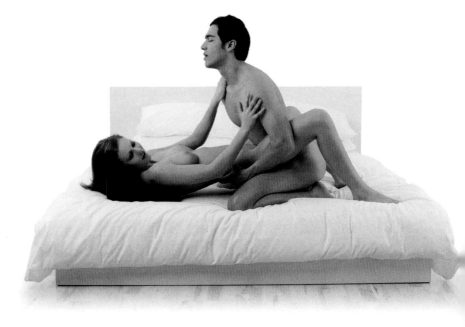

Tonight: He starts with a bang by pulling her hard on to his rod.

Sweet passion: He leans in to feel her body close to his.
Wild passion: He blows her mind with his frantic hip thrusts.

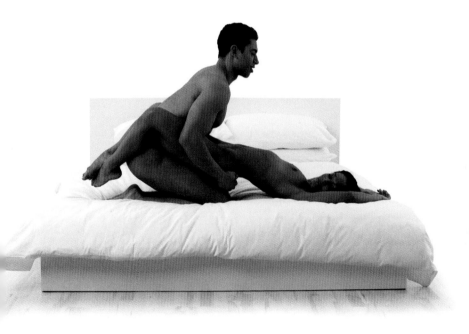

Tonight: You limber up with some sexy moves before the main event.

Clean passion: She stretches out while he slides her up his ramp-like thighs.
Kinky passion: He gives her a wink, then ties her wrists to the bedposts.

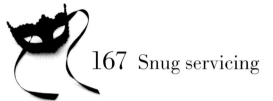

167 Snug servicing

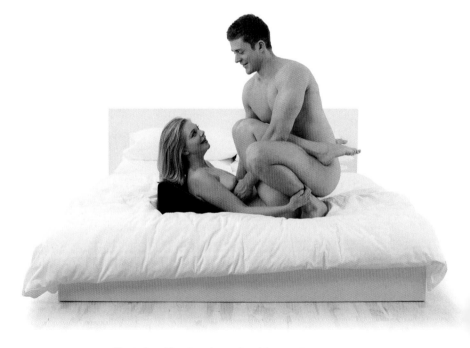

Tonight: He gives her a lewd lesson in compact sex.

Clean passion: He makes her comfortable with wedges and pillows.
Kinky passion: You do it somewhere that you really shouldn't.

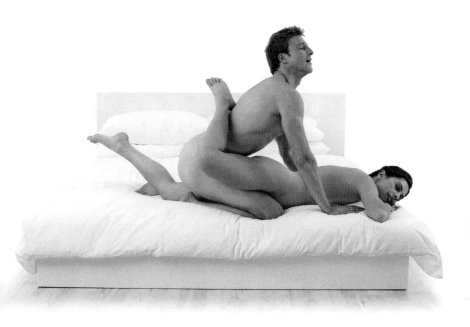

Tonight: He embarks on an anal adventure.

Beginner passion: First, he turns her to putty with his tongue.
Sexpert passion: She relaxes fully, and glides back on to him.

169 Side-splitting delights

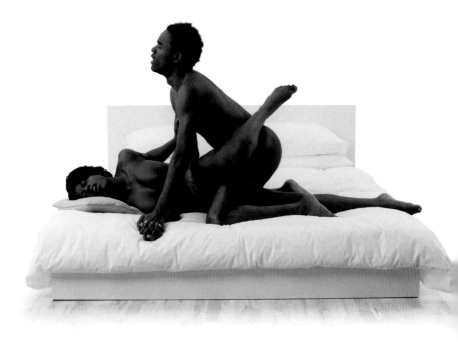

Tonight: He makes it a session of novel angles and piercing penetration.

Sweet passion: He makes her dissolve with gentle belly strokes.
Wild passion: He raises her leg in the air, and goes in deep.

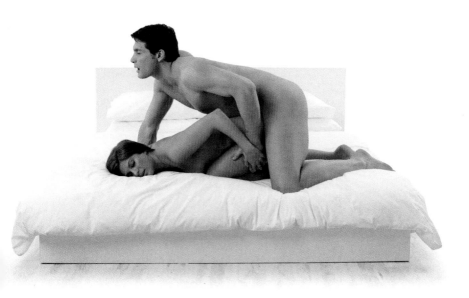

Tonight: She curls up, and invites him through the back door.

Beginner passion: He enjoys a slow dance with her.
Sexpert passion: He glides in, and boogies the night away.

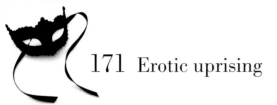

171 Erotic uprising

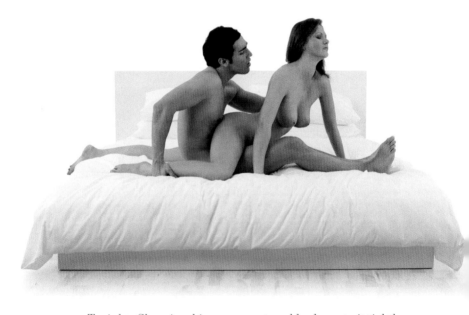

Tonight: She seizes his monument, and backs on to it tightly.

Clean passion: She doesn't surrender her position until dawn.
Kinky passion: She makes him smolder by withdrawing at the 11th hour.

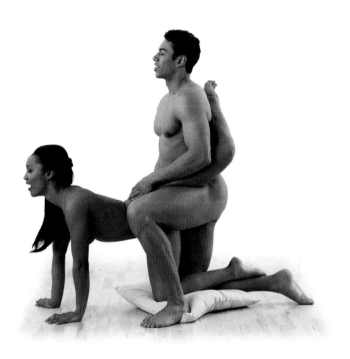

Tonight: You indulge in a night of doggie sex—with flourishes.

Sweet passion: She turns to look at him as she reaches her peak.
Wild passion: She moans one-word orders: "Harder," "Faster," "Deeper.".

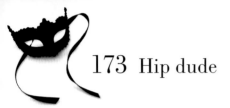

173 Hip dude

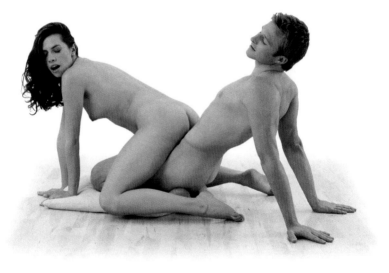

Tonight: He shows her his hip-thrusting magic.

Quickie passion: He gyrates like Elvis.
Lingering passion: He cools the tempo with slow undulations.

Sweet doggie 174

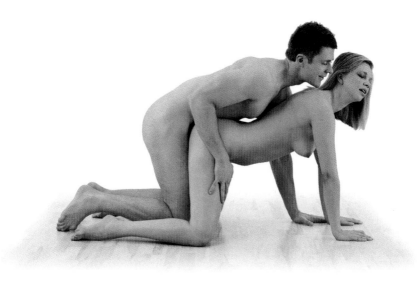

Tonight: He takes her through the tender versions of this classic position.

Fun passion: He growls amorously in her ear.
Fervent passion: She buckles with joy as he makes a super-slow entrance.

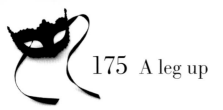

175 A leg up

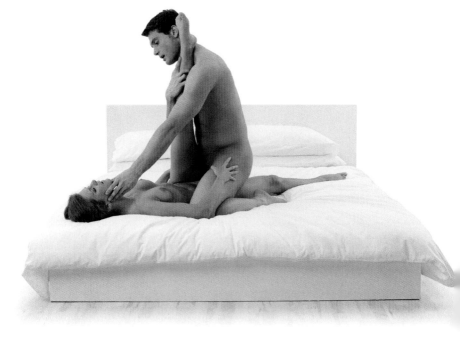

Tonight: She strikes the poses that show off her gorgeous legs.

Sweet passion: He lavishes her legs with caresses.
Wild passion: She blows his mind with sexy stockings and killer heels.

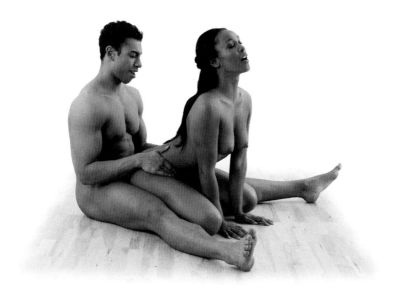

Tonight: He tempts her with the promise of a "sensual massage."

Fun passion: He discovers a stubborn knot of tension between her legs.
Fervent passion: She's so consumed by lust that she slips on to his love muscle.

177 Floating in air

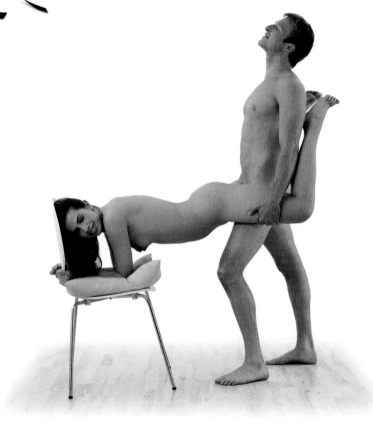

Tonight: He makes sure that her feet don't touch the ground.

Clean passion: He gives her a sturdy chair to rest on.
Kinky passion: He straps her into a sex swing, and makes her fly.

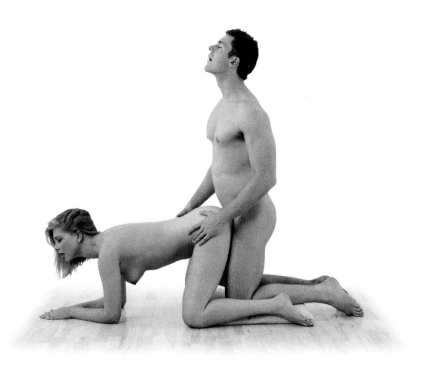

Tonight: He takes her squarely from behind while she's on all fours.

Sweet passion: He puts a rug under her to prevent knee burns.
Wild passion: He hangs on to her shoulders for support.

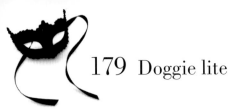

179 Doggie lite

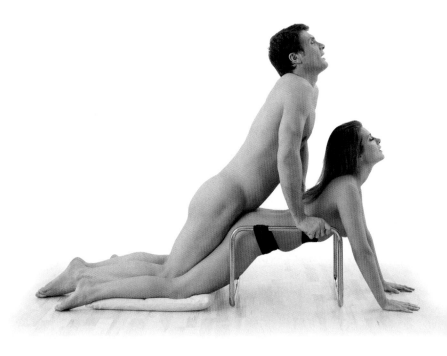

Tonight: He delights in rear-entry positions that she can sustain all night.

Beginner passion: You close your eyes and savor the sensation.
Sexpert passion: You get off by watching yourselves in a mirror.

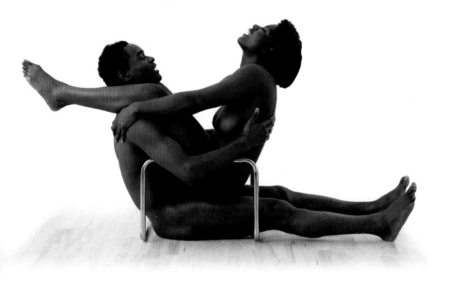

Tonight: He goes to heaven by bouncing her up and down on a sex chair.

Sweet passion: You talk tenderly to each other before the bouncing bit.
Wild passion: You achieve a velocity that you didn't think possible.

181 Racy rebound

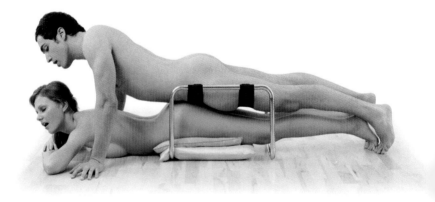

Tonight: He does a push-up on a sex chair, and asks her to slip underneath.

Quickie passion: He ricochets off her body as if there's no tomorrow.
Lingering passion: He stays still, and drives her wild by flexing his love stick.

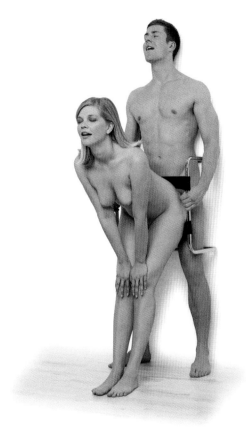

Tonight: He stands firm, ready for an erotic session of all things anal.

Beginner passion: She's in charge of the speed and the depth.
Sexpert passion: She bends over at a 90-degree angle, and he's in all the way.

183 Getting into the groove

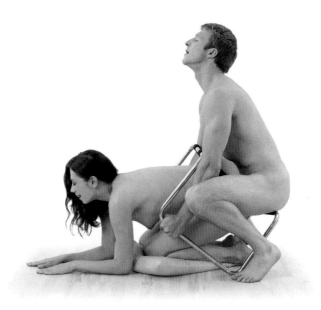

Tonight: He finds the right angle, and settles into a sexy, thrusting groove.

Fun passion: You move in time to fast dance music.
Fervent passion: You move to a funky and soulful tune.

Depth charge 184

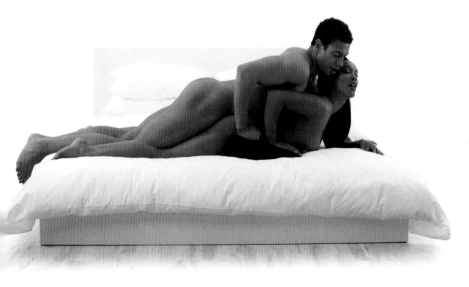

Tonight: He gives her shock waves by penetrating her deeply from behind.

Beginner passion: He thrusts, then stays still for her sensual pleasure.
Sexpert passion: He thrusts using a rhythmic pattern... all night long.

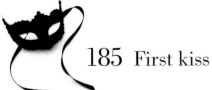

185 First kiss

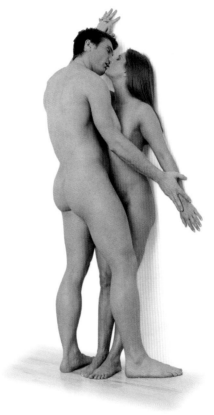

Tonight: He kisses her like it is the first time.

Clean passion: He stops to let her breathe.
Kinky passion: He presses her hard against the wall, and bites her lip.

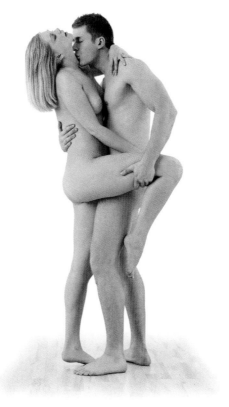

Tonight: He starts by showering her with ravenous kisses.

Quickie passion: You fall to the floor, and get down to business.
Lingering passion: You keep yourselves busy with an intense snog.

187 Romantic night in

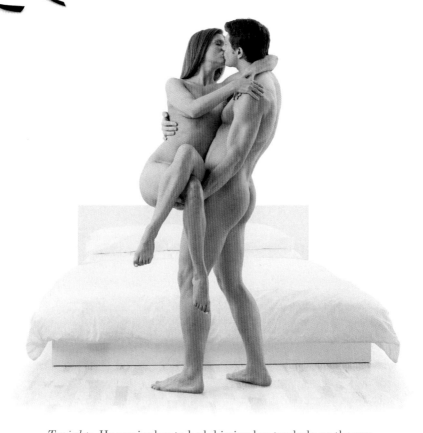

Tonight: He carries her to bed, kissing her tenderly on the way.

Clean passion: He's transformed the bedroom into an erotic haven.
Kinky passion: He's got a box of X-rated toys under the bed.

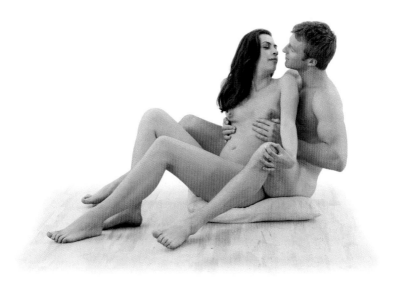

Tonight: He prolongs that pre-kiss moment until she's weak with lust.

Fun passion: He brushes his lips with hers, then pulls away.
Fervent passion: He can't wait, and pushes his tongue softly into her mouth.

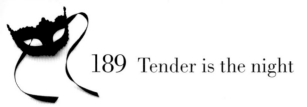

189 Tender is the night

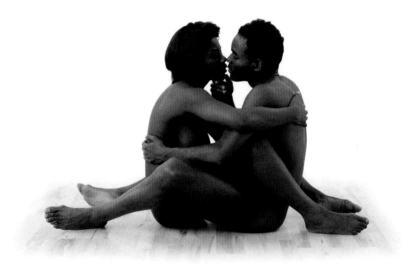

Tonight: You sit smoochily close, and inhale each other's fragrance.

Sweet passion: He smiles before he kisses her tenderly.
Wild passion: You snog with first-time fervor.

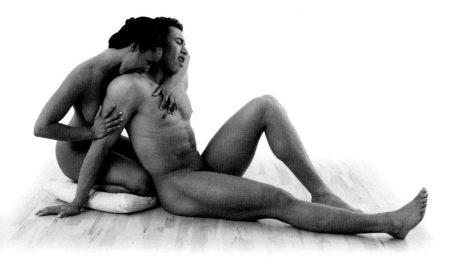

Tonight: She pounces and threatens to eat him all up.

Quickie passion: She bites him into submission, then has her way with him.
Lingering passion: She spends the night nibbling and nuzzling his body.

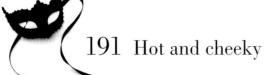

191 Hot and cheeky

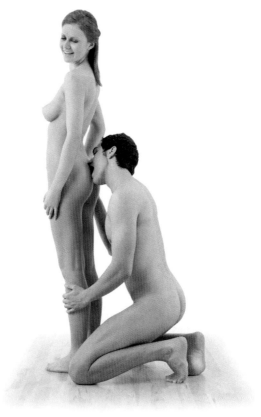

Tonight: He lavishes her butt with steamy oral attention.

Clean passion: He cruises her mounds with soft lips and tongue.
Kinky passion: He brings her to her knees with hard, hungry nips.

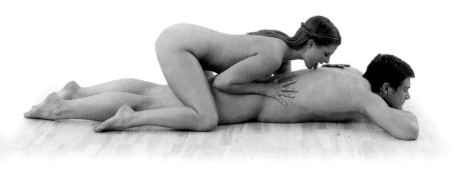

Tonight: She makes him writhe with her sharp, pointy tongue.

Quickie passion: She flips him over, and flicks her tongue on his serpent.
Lingering passion: She takes a languorous licking tour along his back.

193 Toe tantalizer

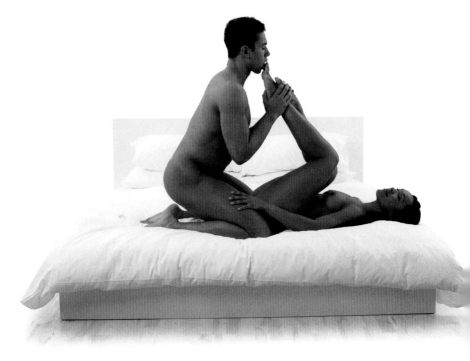

Tonight: He worships her feet with his lips, teeth, and tongue.

Fun passion: He gives each toe individual attention.
Fervent passion: He kisses her soles as ardently as he'd kiss her lips.

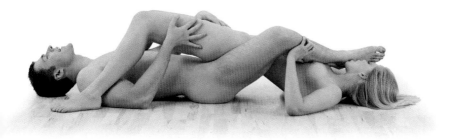

Tonight: You add intense frisson to sex by sensually licking his feet.

Beginner passion: She darts her tongue between his toes.
Sexpert passion: She takes his toes in her teeth, and knows how hard to bite.

195 Rude interruption

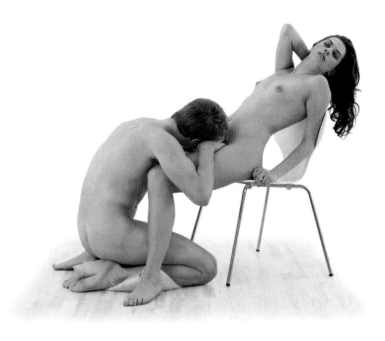

Tonight: He gives her a persuasive reason to stop work.

Fun passion: She bites her lip, and tries to carry on.
Fervent passion: She drops everything, and slides to the edge of her chair.

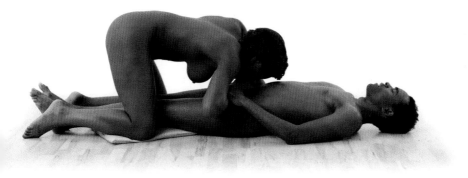

Tonight: He lies back while she sculpts his rock skillfully.

Quickie passion: She's keen to finish the job to his satisfaction.
Lingering passion: She sits back to admire her erotic artwork.

197 Sunday night special

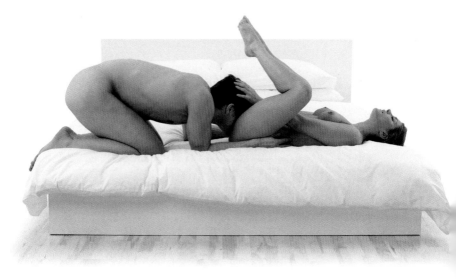

Tonight: He starts the week by heading down south.

Clean passion: He asks if she's comfortable before he begins.
Kinky passion: She grabs his hair, and brazenly moves his head.

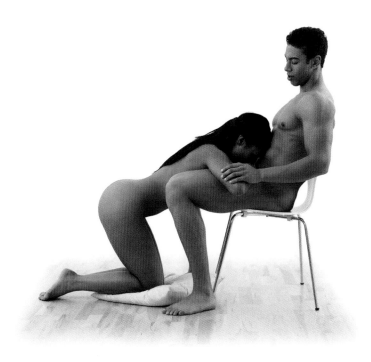

Tonight: She pays homage to his wand by burying her face in his lap.

Sweet passion: She steams him up with her hot breath on his tip.
Wild passion: She slides her lips all the way down to his base, and up again.

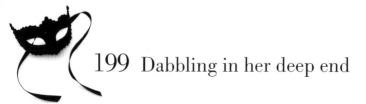

199 Dabbling in her deep end

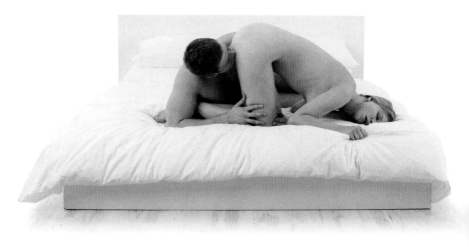

Tonight: He sets the tone with some naughty tongue dabbling.

Fun passion: He keeps his tongue still while she wiggles.
Fervent passion: She pushes herself deliriously into his face.

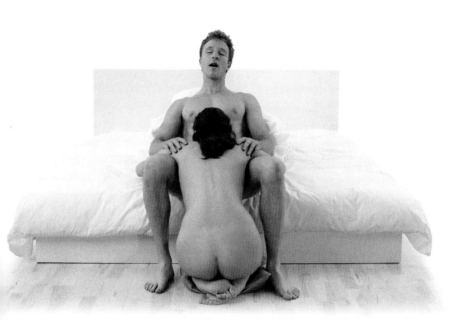

Tonight: She marks the occasion with some awesome oral.

Beginner passion: She concentrates on constant motion.
Sexpert passion: She gazes up at him adoringly as she moves.

201 Feast night

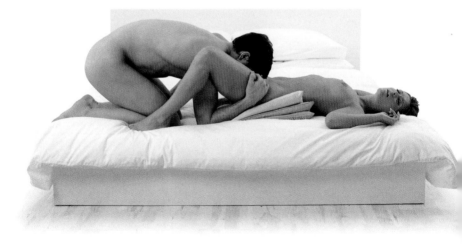

Tonight: He treats her body as if it's a bawdy banquet table.

Clean passion: He drinks champagne from her navel.
Kinky passion: He slides a cucumber inside her.

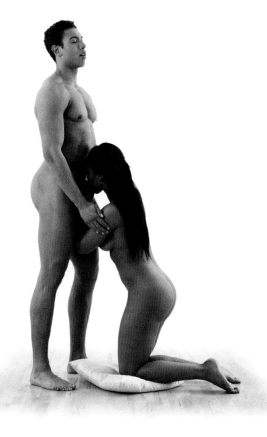

Tonight: She kneels before him, and takes him firmly in hand and mouth.

Clean passion: She slinks up his body for a lust-fueled kiss.
Kinky passion: She pulls away at the heavenly moment so he can anoint her.

203 One night in heaven

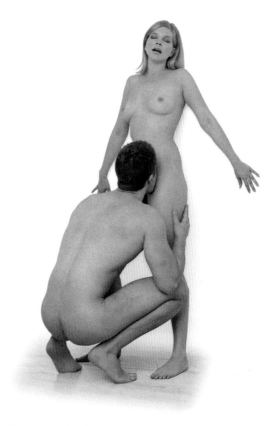

Tonight: He presses his lips to her pearl, and says he's staying there.

Beginner passion: He turns her to liquid with licks, lunges, and laps.
Sexpert passion: He adds some G-spot handiwork to make her delirious.

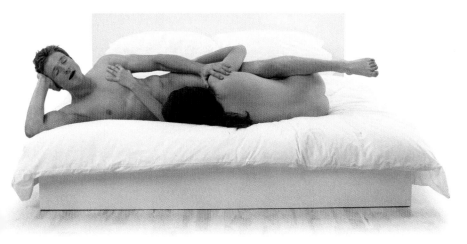

Tonight: She offers him a BJ session in which he sets the pace.

Clean passion: He sighs softly, and thrusts his hips gently.
Kinky passion: He groans deeply, and moves her head firmly.

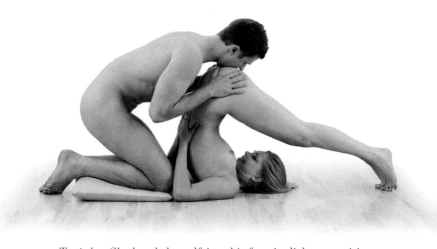

Tonight: She bends herself into his favorite lick-me positions.

Beginner passion: He glides his tongue over her buttocks and thighs.
Sexpert passion: He probes her back garden with his tongue.

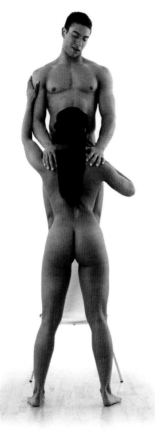

Tonight: He takes an elevated approach to oral sex.

Quickie passion: He paces her by moving his hips in rhythm with her lips.
Lingering passion: She draws delicate lines with the tip of her tongue.

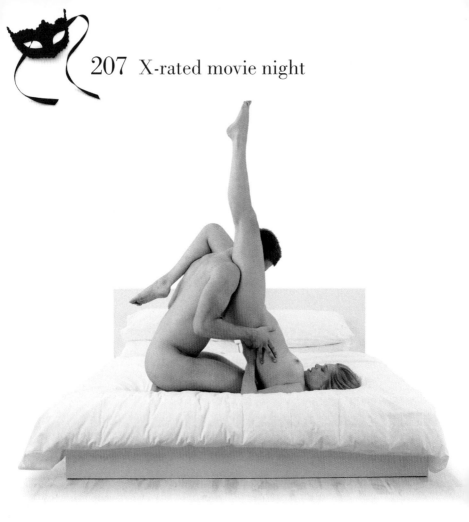

207 X-rated movie night

Tonight: You film yourselves performing lush acts in sexy poses.

Clean passion: You go for artistic long shots.
Kinky passion: You invite a friend over to take some hand-held close-ups.

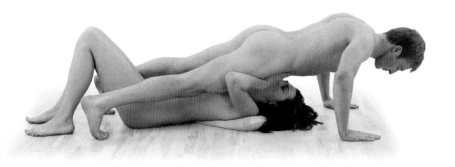

Tonight: She studies his main part until she's lip perfect.

Fun passion: He does push-ups into her mouth.
Fervent passion: She makes him tremble with her intense performance.

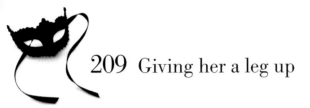

209 Giving her a leg up

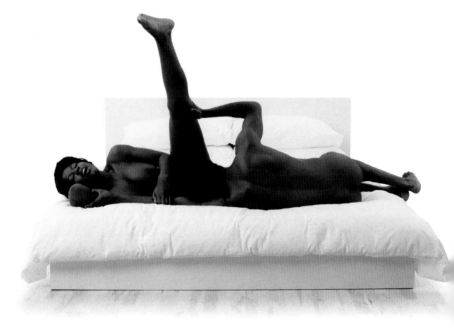

Tonight: He lies head-to-crotch, and opens her up to intimate ecstasy.

Clean passion: He tickles her inner thighs.
Kinky passion: He gets face-in, and uses his teeth as well as his tongue.

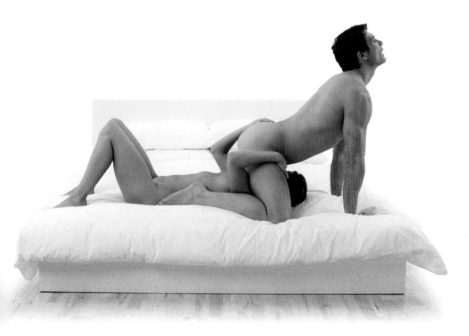

Tonight: She heads down to attend a very private view.

Clean passion: She puts a peppermint in her mouth to make him zing.
Kinky passion: He watches an explosively erotic movie.

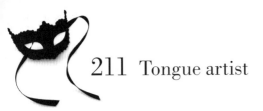

211 Tongue artist

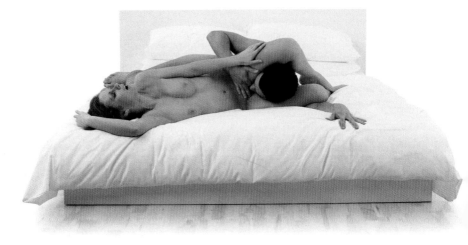

Tonight: He sneaks between her legs to begin his masterpiece.

Sweet passion: He signs his name with the tip of his tongue.
Wild passion: He makes her wet and glossy with bold brushstrokes.

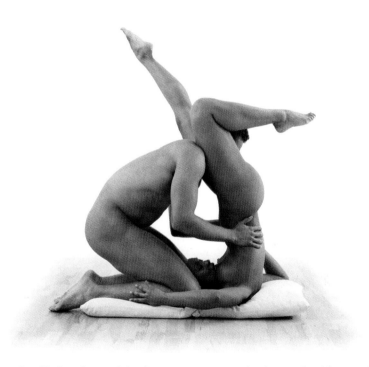

Tonight: He laps her with his burning tongue as she does a shoulder-stand.

Beginner passion: He lovingly clasps her back, and shoulders her thighs.
Sexpert passion: He makes her swoon by sweeping her up into an upright 69.

213 Ecstasy heights

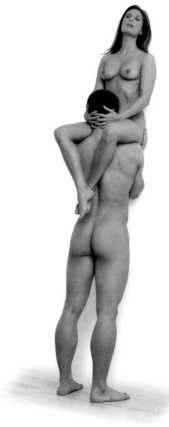

Tonight: He makes her night with the highest form of flattery.

Sweet passion: He promises not to let her go.
Wild passion: He slides her down until she lands on his tower..

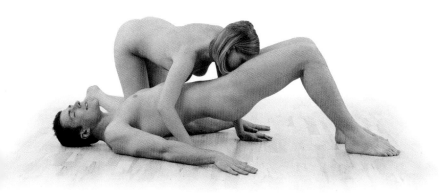

Tonight: She goes on a truffle hunt along his naked body.

Clean passion: She stops for regular tastings.
Kinky passion: She tries teabagging him.

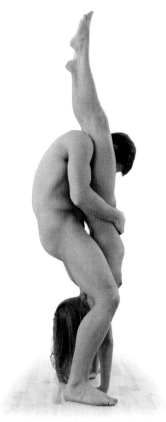

Tonight: You form stunning sculptures as you lick each other.

Beginner passion: You practice privately in the bedroom.
Sexpert passion: You throw a sex party and perform live.

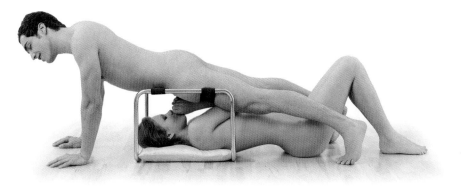

Tonight: She uses her hands, mouth, and a sex chair to tackle his plumbing.

Quickie passion: Her hot hands and twisty tongue make him overflow.
Lingering passion: She pulls back when she feels his pressure rising.

217 Sex whispering

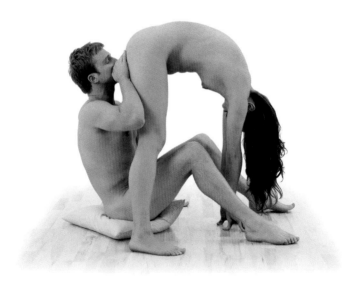

Tonight: He reads her secrets with his hands, lips, and tongue.

Sweet passion: He guesses what she wants, and delivers it.
Wild passion: He brings her to the floor with his intense talents.

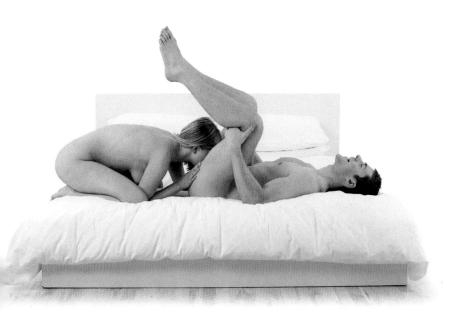

Tonight: She spends the night befriending his twins.

Sweet passion: She delights him with barely there licks.
Wild passion: She gives him a feverish tongue-lashing.

219 Mischievous mechanic

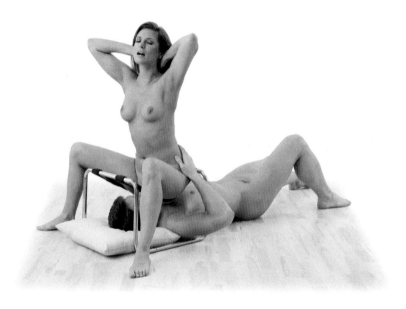

Tonight: He slides underneath to give her a saucy servicing.

Quickie passion: He gets her engine going immediately.
Lingering passion: He starts by stroking her bodywork.

Deep throat 220

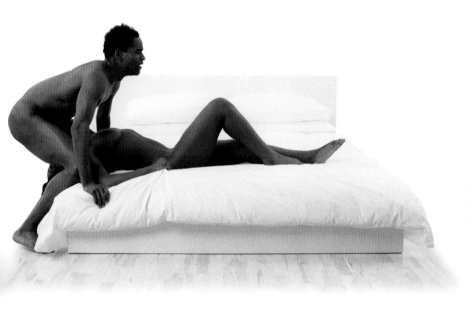

Tonight: She throws her head back, and swallows him whole.

Beginner passion: She practices on a cucumber first.
Sexpert passion: She gets super-aroused, and takes him in bit by bit.

221 Lazy wheelbarrow

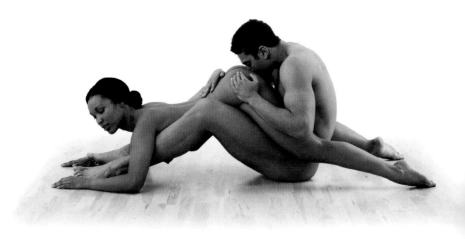

Tonight: He tends her garden with his tongue.

Fun passion: He makes her lickably sweet with strawberry lube.
Fervent passion: He gives himself up to moans of feverish desire.

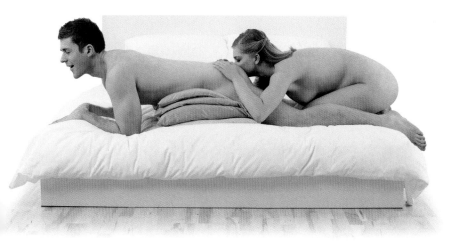

Tonight: She blows off his manhole cover, and licks him into shape.

Quickie passion: He pumps hard into some pillows.
Lingering passion: She inspects all of his man bits—one bit at a time.

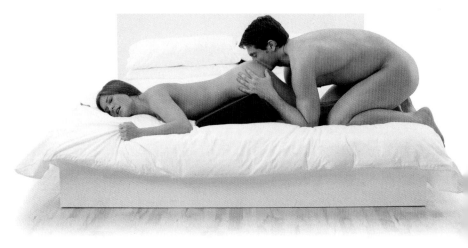

Tonight: He gives her one hot, sheet-clenching experience after another.

Clean passion: He tongues her cheeks.
Kinky passion: He dives deep into her groove.

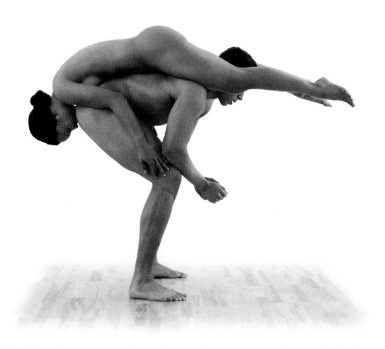

Tonight: She rests on him, and twirls her tongue on the star of his show.

Quickie passion: She does some fast and fancy handiwork on his front stage.
Lingering passion: You spend the night inventing kinky new licking poses.

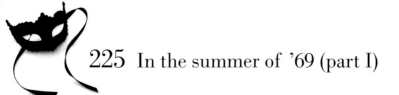

225 In the summer of '69 (part I)

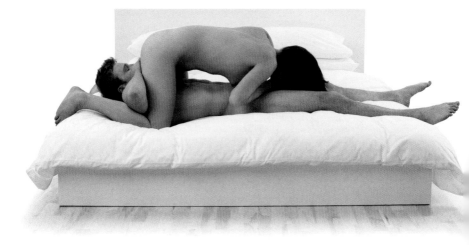

Tonight: You succumb to a hot, balmy evening of languorous licking.

Beginner passion: You take breaks to cool off.
Sexpert passion: You roll over halfway through, so that she's underneath.

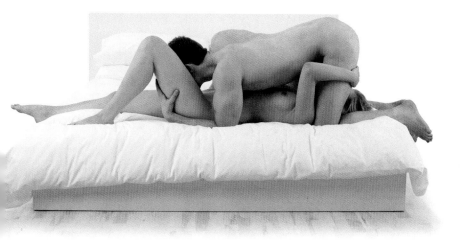

Tonight: You get down to business, and shake your heads vigorously.

Sweet passion: He adopts a ladies-first policy.
Wild passion: You get carried away, and writhe like animals.

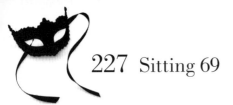

227 Sitting 69

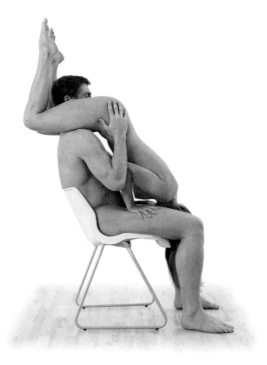

Tonight: She dives between his legs, and he dives between hers.

Quickie passion: You suck, flick, and twirl with abandon.
Lingering passion: This is just the starting position.

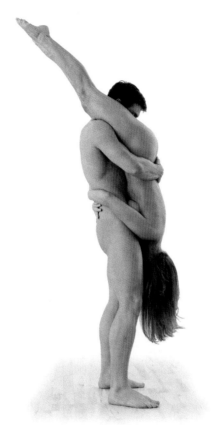

Tonight: He holds her in a tight clinch as you do the double kiss.

Fun passion: You try talking with your mouth full.
Fervent passion: You sink feverishly to the floor to continue in comfort.

229 Floating 69—for her

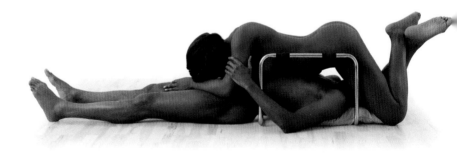

Tonight: She lets a sex chair take the strain to explore each other's best bits.

Beginner passion: She wiggles around for perfect mouth-genital impact.
Sexpert passion: She uses her knees to set up a delirious rhythm.

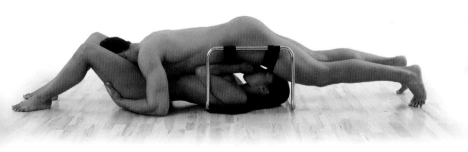

Tonight: You swap over, so that he can deliver some floating oral.

Sweet passion: You start by delivering slow, luscious kisses.
Wild passion: She grabs his ass, and bounces him in and out.

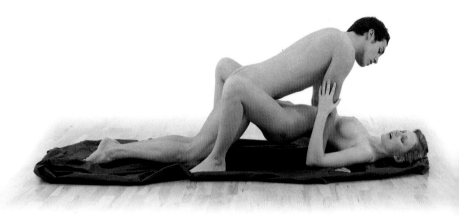

Tonight: She delights him with a series of hip-fluttering moves.

Quickie passion: She flutters feverishly.
Lingering passion: She flutters fleetingly.

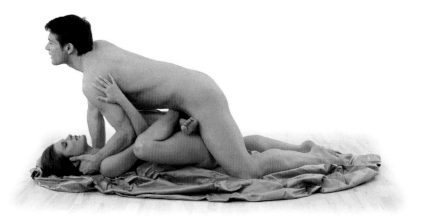

Tonight: You discover the Eastern art of yoga-style sex.

Sweet passion: You meditate on the energy flowing between you.
Wild passion: She puts her feet behind her head in plow pose.

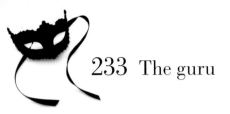

233 The guru

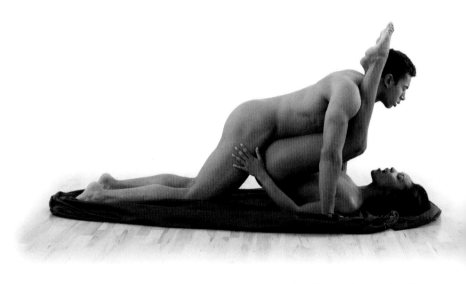

Tonight: He starts in missionary, then eases her legs higher and higher.

Beginner passion: You save this one for those peak-lust moments.
Sexpert passion: You do it this way all night long.

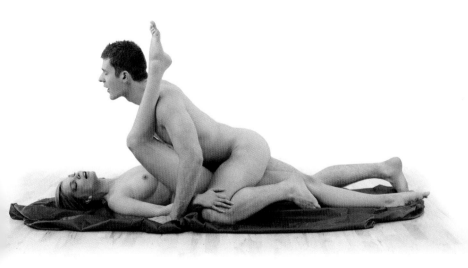

Tonight: He gives her ecstatic split-up-the-middle feelings.

Quickie passion: You gasp and pant your way to a shuddering O.
Lingering passion: You take deep, slow, sensual belly breaths.

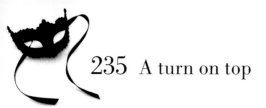

235 A turn on top

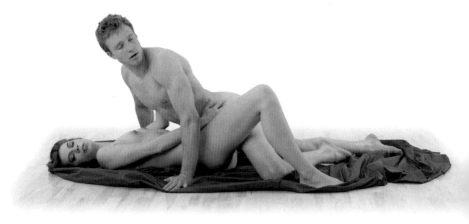

Tonight: He tries the ancient erotic ritual of turning 180 degrees during sex.

Beginner passion: He takes breaks to revive his erection.
Sexpert passion: He spins effortlessly with a raging hard-on.

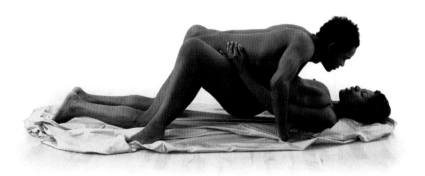

Tonight: He stays still while she rises up for an amorous meeting.

Fun passion: She drives him crazy by hovering on his tip.
Fervent passion: She sticks close in an intensely erotic tryst.

237 Garden of paradise

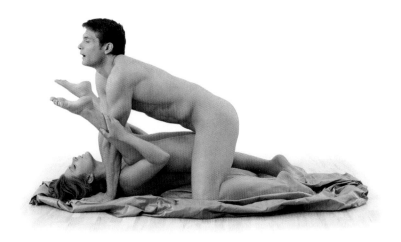

Tonight: He plunges joyously into her lush garden.

Quickie passion: He can't help but sprinkle his seed.
Lingering passion: He wanders slowly among her flowers.

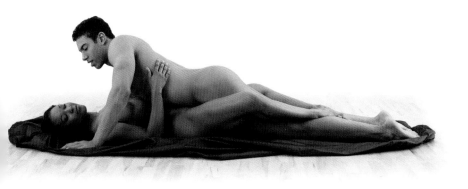

Tonight: She welcomes him aboard for a smoochy start to the evening.

Fun passion: She gives him a naughty look, and asks for a kiss.
Fervent passion: He melts into her with an ecstatic "mmmmmm".

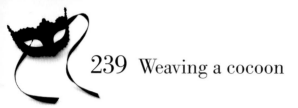

239 Weaving a cocoon

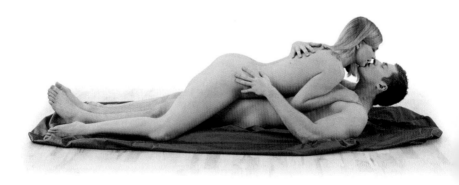

Tonight: She slides on to his body, and encloses him in lust.

Sweet passion: She basks in his sensual heat.
Wild passion: She wriggles, writhes, and jiggles on top of him.

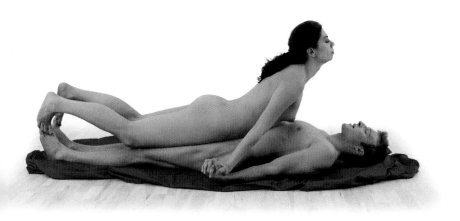

Tonight: She balances on top, and takes off from his runway.

Quickie passion: He grabs her hips, and makes things turbulent.
Lingering passion: She's on a long haul, and cruises smoothly.

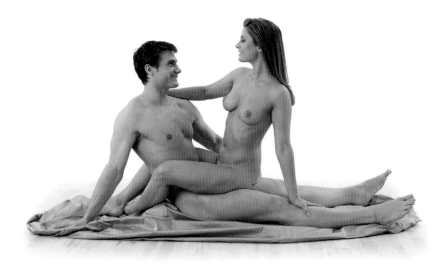

Tonight: She climbs on to his lap, and twines her legs around him.

Beginner passion: She holds him in a titillatingly tight monkey grip.
Sexpert passion: He clasps her close and stands up.

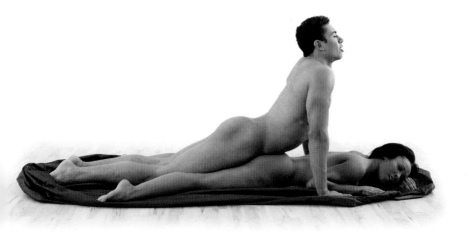

Tonight: He sinks his mighty trunk into her as she lies on her belly.

Quickie passion: He stampedes his way to a bellowing climax.
Lingering passion: He moves inside her with a side-to-side swaying motion.

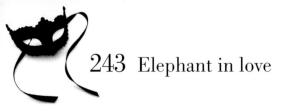

243 Elephant in love

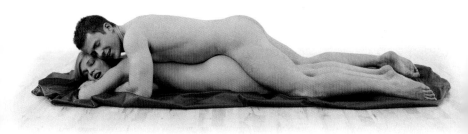

Tonight: He snuggles against her back, and grazes on her shoulders.

Clean passion: He makes this her sexy wake-up call.
Kinky passion: He visits her front watering hole, then her back.

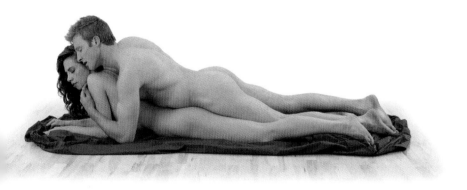

Tonight: You begin with a bedtime hug…

Quickie passion: He uses his position to go in fast and deep.
Lingering passion: He makes her glow with soft caresses.

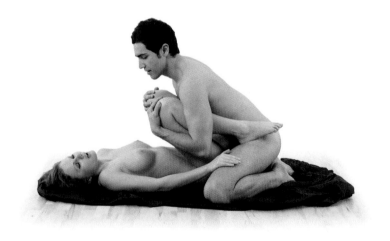

245 Crab's position

Tonight: He treats her to an intimate interlude as he enters from on top.

Fun passion: He hugs her knees playfully.
Fervent passion: He caresses her breasts earnestly.

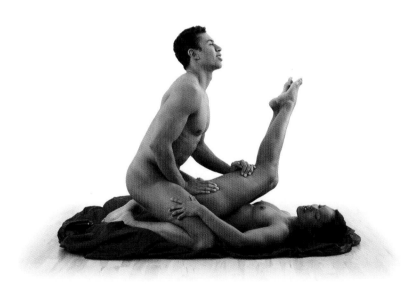

Tonight: He delves deeply into her cave at the climax of an amorous night.

Clean passion: He kisses the soles of her feet tenderly.
Kinky passion: He delivers a resounding spank to the top of her thigh.

247 Heavenly congress

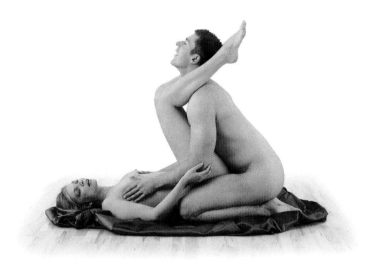

Tonight: You both taste heaven as she slides her legs over his shoulders.

Quickie passion: He channels fast vibrations through her pelvis.
Lingering passion: You meditate on the divine sensations.

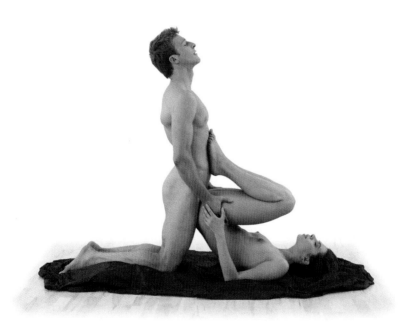

Tonight: You experiment to find the position that takes you highest.

Beginner passion: He offers two firm, supporting hands.
Sexpert passion: She shows off by resting her toes behind her head.

249 Plunge pool

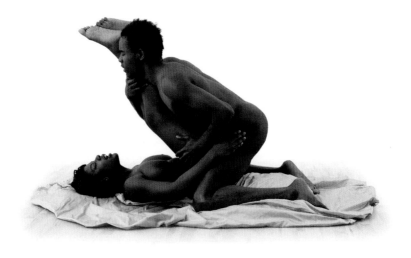

Tonight: He hugs her legs to his body, and plumbs her depths.

Fun passion: He compliments her on the suppleness of her groin.
Fervent passion: He rocks her to a slow, but shattering climax.

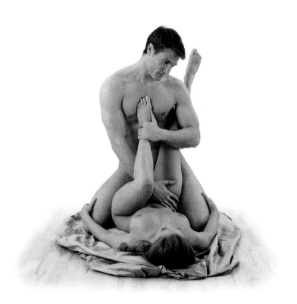

Tonight: He makes her night special with soft, shimmery touches.

Quickie passion: He goes straight to work with his silkworm.
Lingering passion: He draws her slowly into his cocoon.

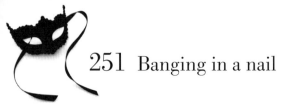

251 Banging in a nail

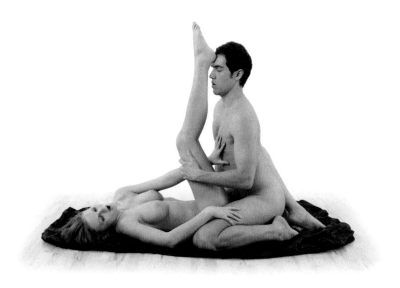

Tonight: You start here, then work through the *Kama Sutra* classics.

Fun passion: She tries to keep her foot on his forehead when he comes.

Fervent passion: You stay still, and share a moment of erotic bonding.

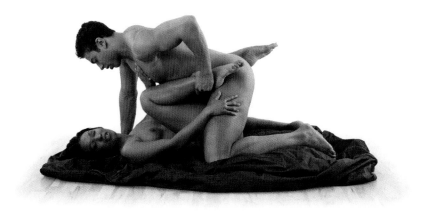

Tonight: He shows her what he's made of with a series of galloping moves.

Sweet passion: She reaches up, and touches his lips with her fingertips.
Wild passion: He pushes her knees up high, and races home.

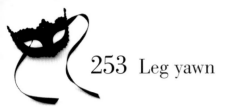

253 Leg yawn

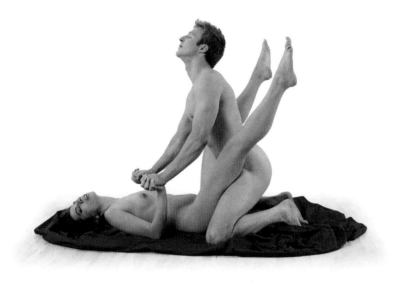

Tonight: She kicks off the evening with a *Kama Sutra* favorite.

Fun passion: She playfully raps his butt with her heels.
Fervent passion: She uses her feet to pull him blissfully close.

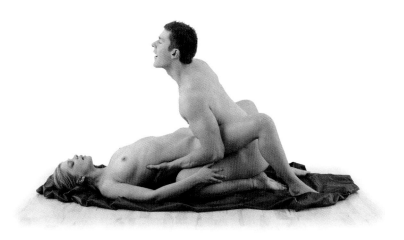

Tonight: She lies back as he plunges his swelling into her ocean.

Sweet passion: She smiles at him as pleasure ripples through her.
Wild passion: He makes his moves rough and choppy.

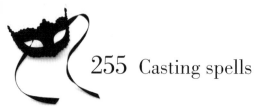

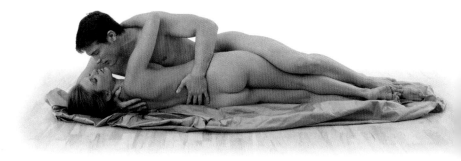

Tonight: You share an evening of spellbinding love.

Quickie passion: You let yourselves be overwhelmed.
Lingering passion: You allow the magic to unfold.

Tong position 256

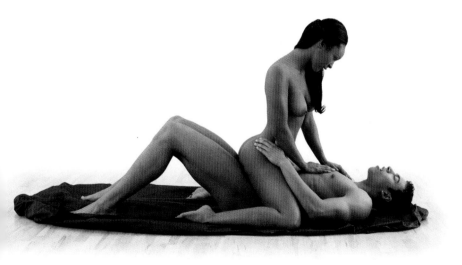

Tonight: She makes him swoon by sliding down his thighs on to his tool.

Beginner passion: She makes him smile by squeezing him with her Kegels.
Sexpert passion: She makes him gasp with her tong-like grip.

257 Wild abandon

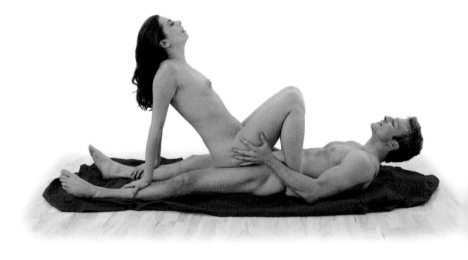

Tonight: You throw your heads back as you abandon yourselves to lust.

Fun passion: Try it lying under a mirrored ceiling.
Fervent passion: You do it outdoors, and see stars.

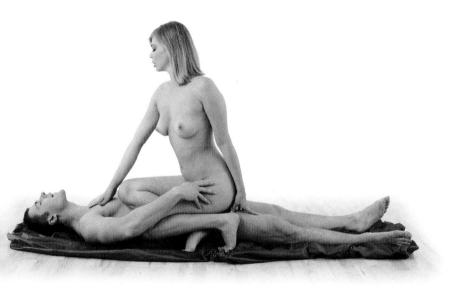

Tonight: She impales herself on his toy, then spins around 360 degrees.

Beginner passion: She opts for an easier 180-degree twist.
Sexpert passion: She goes full circle, stopping for regular thrust breaks.

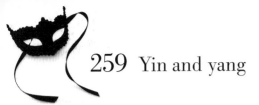

259 Yin and yang

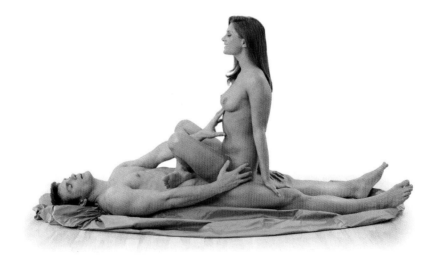

Tonight: You spend the night harmonizing your sexual energies.

Clean passion: You sensually merge as if one.
Kinky passion: She grinds his yang raw.

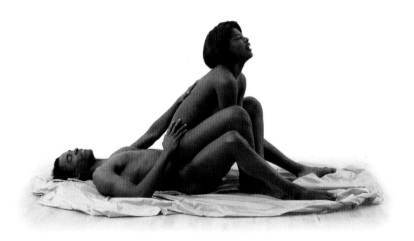

Tonight: He takes a laid-back approach while she sits perkily on top.

Fun passion: He looks up, she looks down, and you ogle each other's bits.
Fervent passion: He cries out uncontrollably as he hits the high note.

261 Honeybee

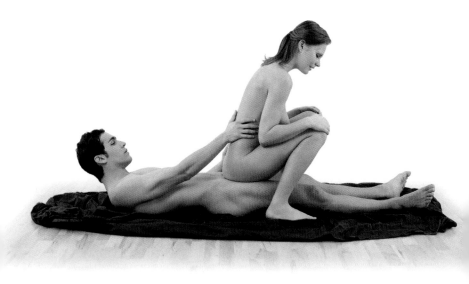

Tonight: She thrills him by sitting on top to suck out his nectar.

Clean passion: She hovers, wiggles, and flies off.
Kinky passion: She buzzes his balls with a fingertip vibrator.

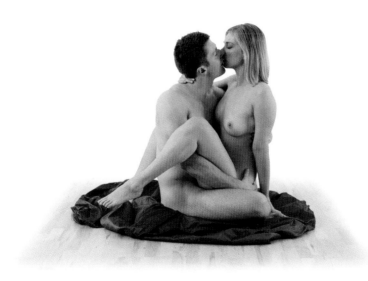

Tonight: You devote yourselves to hot cuddles and super-close sex.

Quickie passion: You dive into each other's arms after weeks apart.
Lingering passion: You make each other wait before soothing the swelling.

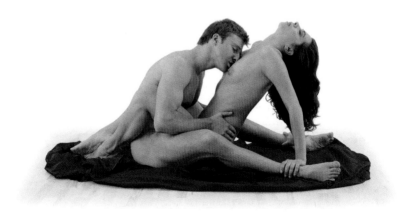

Tonight: You sit for a sizzling session in which neither of you takes the lead.

Sweet passion: You tenderly stroke each other's face.
Wild passion: You kiss madly as he lifts her on to his pole.

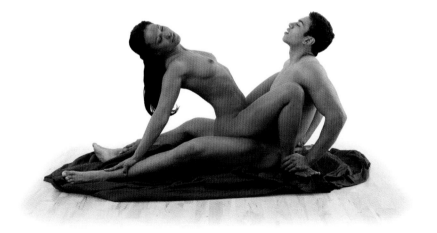

Tonight: You drench each other with desire as you flow into your final pose.

Beginner passion: He announces his jet with a delirious moan.
Sexpert passion: He's primed her G-spot for a gush moment of her own.

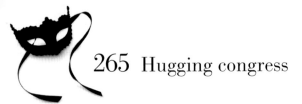

265 Hugging congress

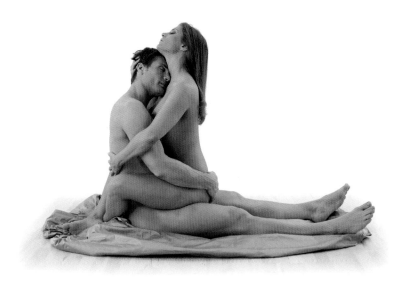

Tonight: You hold each other close and don't let go.

Fun passion: You try falling sideways while you're still joined.
Fervent passion: You sit still, and listen to each other breathe.

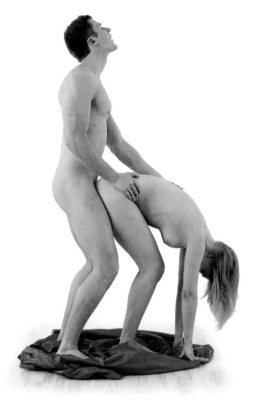

Tonight: You try some of the raunchiest sex positions known to man and beast.

Beginner passion: She rests her forearms on a table, and looks back coyly.
Sexpert passion: She puts her hands down, and pushes her ass up.

267 Hammering in a nail

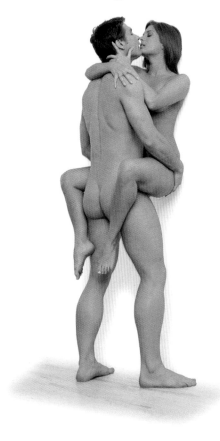

Tonight: He picks her up, and shows off his skillful toolwork.

Clean passion: He chooses a wall that can take the strain.
Kinky passion: You try it on a train or plane for extra jigginess.

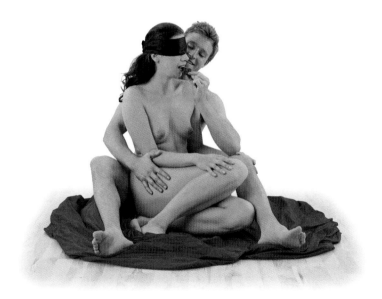

Tonight: He arouses her senses one by one, beginning with taste.

Sweet passion: He slips dark, rich chocolate between her lips.
Wild passion: He embraces her, and kisses champagne into her mouth.

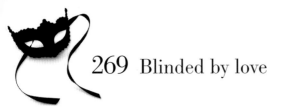

269 Blinded by love

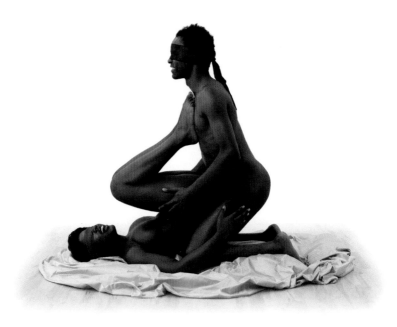

Tonight: You merge in ecstasy as he feels his way in.

Quickie passion: He can't resist the magnetic pull of her front porch.
Lingering passion: First, you explore each other with your fingertips.

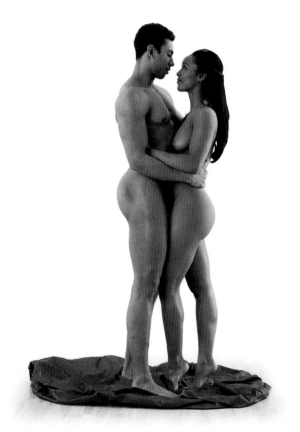

Tonight: You begin with Tantric magic by gazing into each other's eyes.

Fun passion: You wink cheekily, and let the ravishing commence.
Fervent passion: Say: "I honor your body with my heart and soul."

271 A brush with lust

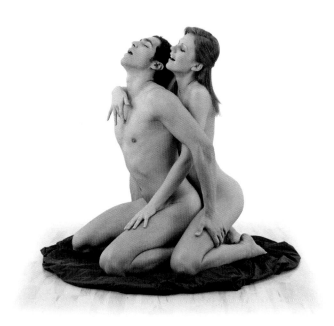

Tonight: She begins by trailing her fingertips longingly over his contours.

Sweet passion: She caresses his neck with her soft, warm lips.
Wild passion: She slides her hands hard and feverishly all over his body.

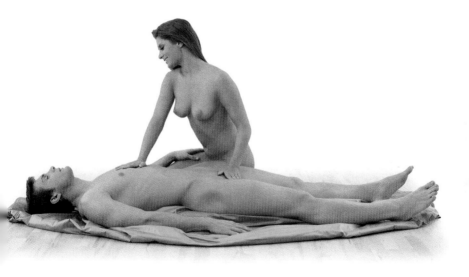

Tonight: She blasts his chakras with fiery sexual energy.

Beginner passion: She presses her palms to his heart and lingam.
Sexpert passion: She unleashes his kundalini with a Tantric massage.

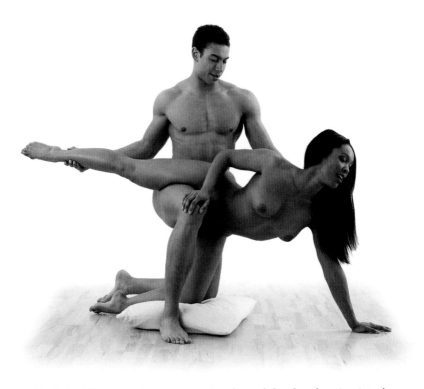

273 Taken by storm

Tonight: He sends pleasure coursing through her by plunging into her.

Quickie passion: He makes thunder roll with darts and flicks of his hips.
Lingering passion: He soothes her storm with long sensual strokes.

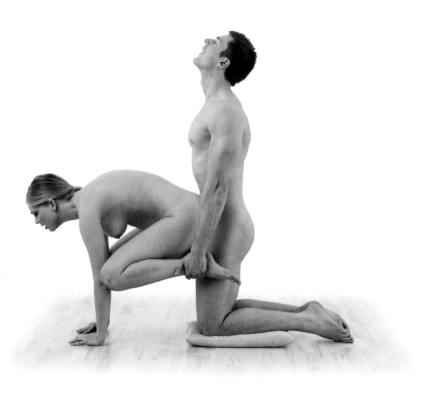

Tonight: You both get high on some super-advanced sex moves.

Clean passion: He's quick and efficient at operating his hydraulics.
Kinky passion: You both wear fetish-style PVC bodysuits.

275 Fiery night

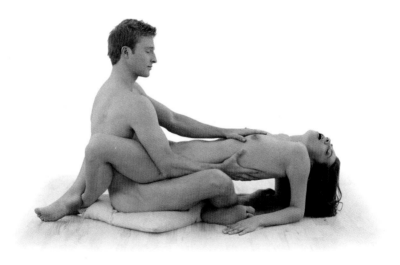

Tonight: You strip off, and get frisky by a roaring fire.

Fun passion: You feed each other toasted marshmallows.
Fervent passion: You give into the heat surging through you.

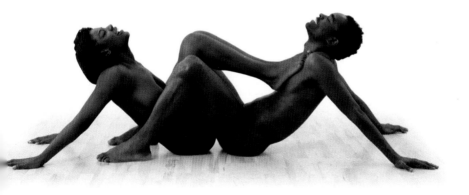

Tonight: You laugh your way to orgasm as you invent erotic entanglements.

Fun passion: You hire a photographer to record the event.
Fervent passion: Your laughter turns into sighs of pleasure.

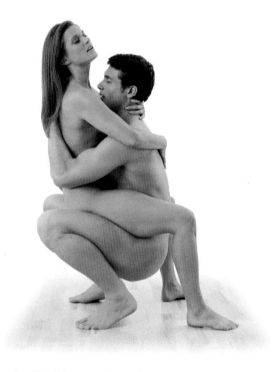

Tonight: You'll try anything that gives you a wobbly thrill.

Beginner passion: You surround yourselves with cushions.
Sexpert passion: He bounces as he balances.

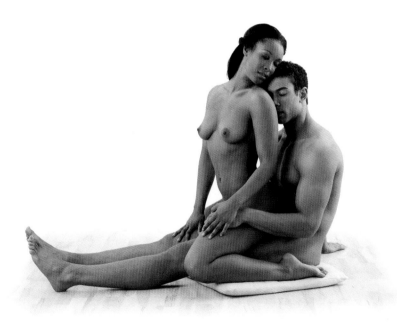

Tonight: You enjoy a series of hop-on, hop-off poses as the sun sets.

Fun passion: You pull the blanket over you, and pretend to be invisible.
Fervent passion: You feed succulent tidbits to each other.

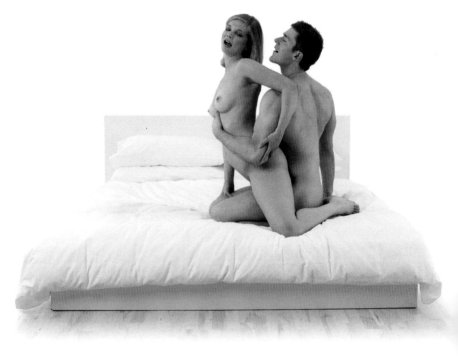

Tonight: He drives her wild by taking her to the edge, and pulling her back.

Clean passion: He holds her firmly as she teeters.
Kinky passion: He makes her beg him to carry on.

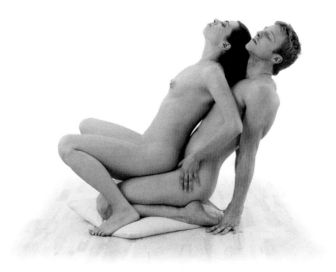

Tonight: Like a gentleman, he offers her the best seat in the house.

Beginner passion: He makes sure that his seat stays sturdy.
Sexpert passion: He caresses all her frontal pleasure zones.

281 Love's tailor

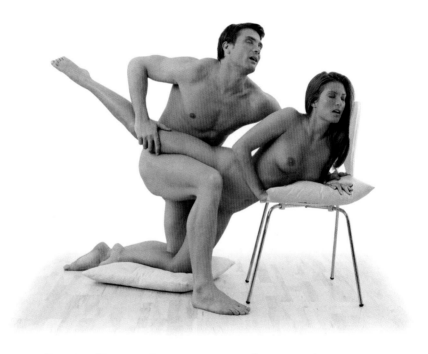

Tonight: She treats him to an evening of sensational scissor moves.

Fun passion: He threads himself into her back buttonhole.
Fervent passion: He presses in deeply for a fit that feels tailor-made.

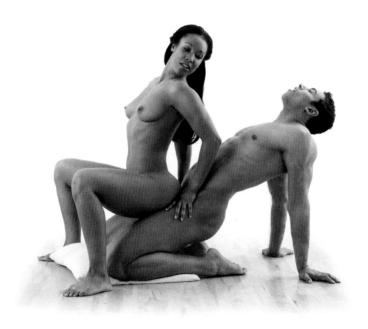

Tonight: She cascades down his front, and impales herself on his rock.

Clean passion: She presses her body to his, and goes with his flow.
Kinky passion: She straddles his face, then slips easily down his front.

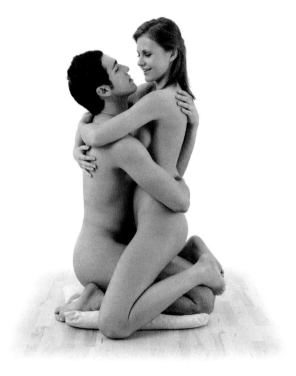

Tonight: You end the evening with a sensual whole-body hug.

Sweet passion: He stays inside her for as long as possible.
Wild passion: He throws her on the floor for Act II.

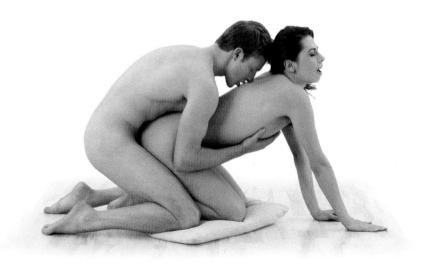

Tonight: She's doing some late-night scrubbing, but he just can't resist.

Beginner passion: You fall to the floor, and go for it.
Sexpert passion: You move up to kitchen-counter sex.

285 Locked in lust

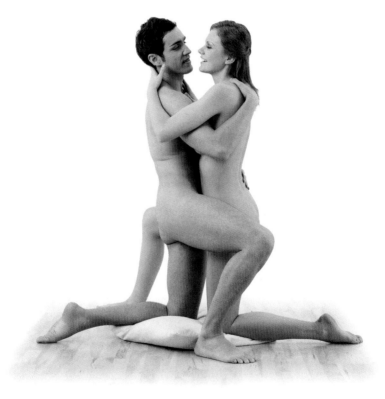

Tonight: You kneel down, and wrap each other in your arms.

Fun passion: You get into a flirty wrestling match.
Fervent passion: You dissolve into a swooning kiss.

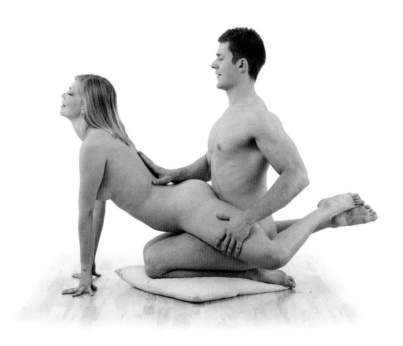

Tonight: He holds her close and delivers a very personal message.

Beginner passion: He gets her tingling by stroking her back.
Sexpert passion: He delivers his message in the bath.

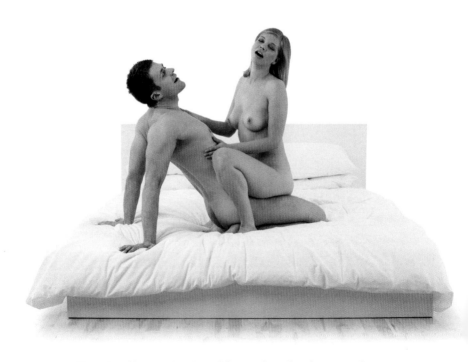

Tonight: She climbs aboard for a ride to her favourite destination.

Fun passion: He provides the rhythm, she provides the sound-effects.
Fervent passion: You lose track of the time, and don't get off until morning.

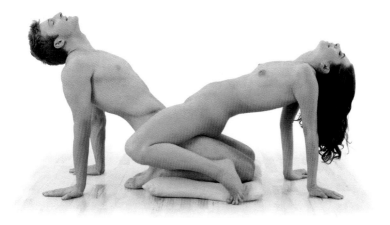

Tonight: She straddles him, and you get into the motion of the ocean.

Beginner passion: She rides his swells, and he caresses her crests.
Sexpert passion: You move as if you're both in a wild storm.

289 The hijack-her

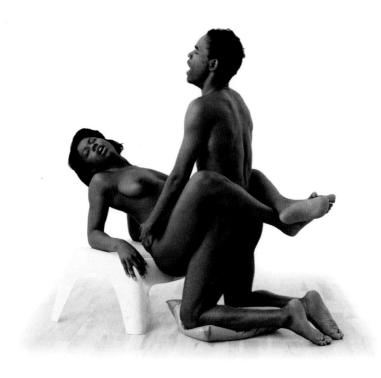

Tonight: He slides her up his body, and makes her an erotic prisoner.

Clean passion: He offers to release her without a ransom.
Lingering passion: He doesn't let her go until you're both spent and dazed.

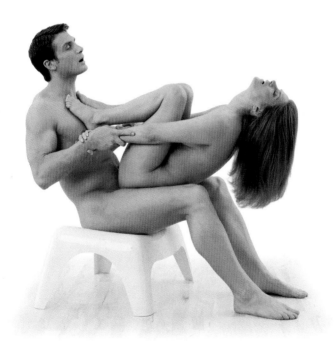

Tonight: He takes her through a series of jet-propelled moves.

Quickie passion: You combust internally within seconds.
Lingering passion: You take sexy refueling breaks.

291 Footstool friskiness

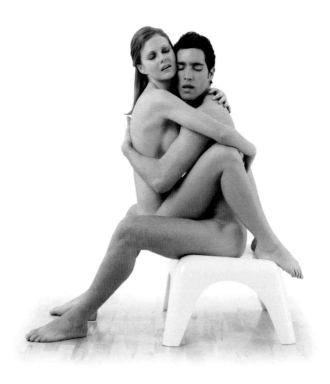

Tonight: You grab the nearest footstool, and get closely entwined.

Sweet passion: You lose yourselves in a time-stopping cuddle.
Wild passion: He picks her up in his arms, and presses her against a wall.

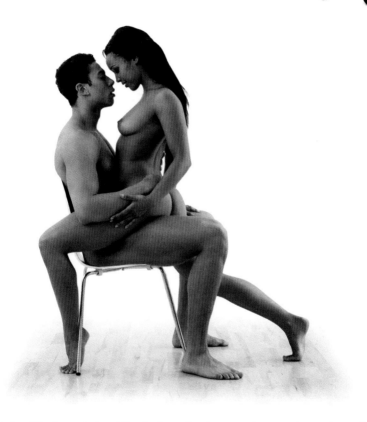

Tonight: He sits quietly while she launches her opening attack warrior-style.

Fun passion: She commands him to unsheathe his sword.
Fervent passion: She declares a truce, and tenderly presses her lips to his.

293 After dinner sins

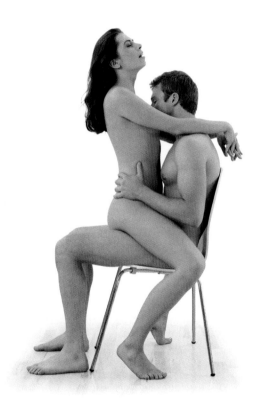

Tonight: She straddles him, and has him for dessert.

Beginner passion: She makes her moves gentle rather than jiggy.
Sexpert passion: She kneels on the floor to sip his liqueur.

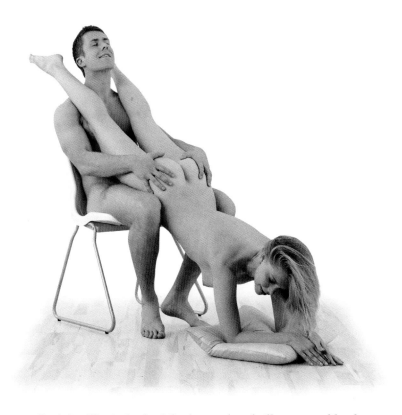

Tonight: He sits back while she gets her thrills at ground level.

Clean passion: He closes his eyes, and squeezes her peaches.
Kinky passion: He reveals an array of naughty spanking tools.

295 Bathroom bliss

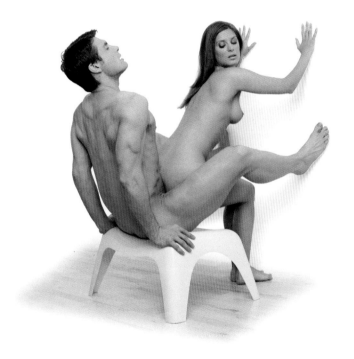

Tonight: Oops, you're accidentally locked in a friend's bathroom.

Sweet passion: You cuddle while you wait to be released.
Wild passion: He flips the toilet seat down and grabs her…

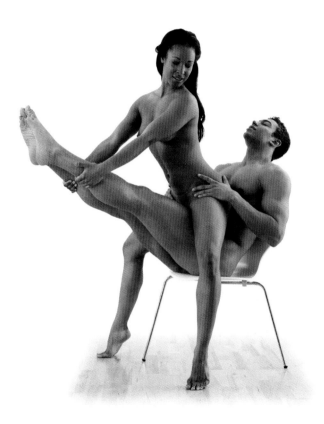

Tonight: He offers to be both horse and riding instructor.

Clean passion: He asks her to practise a light trot or canter.
Kinky passion: He spanks her with a riding crop if she doesn't obey.

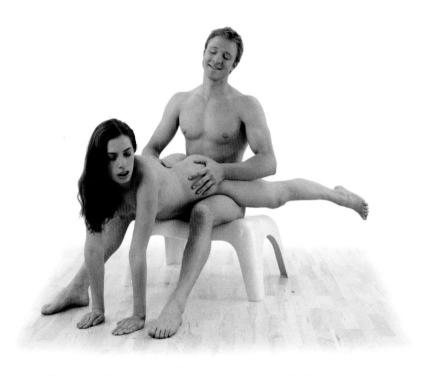

Tonight: He uses fast sawing movements to make her cry out.

Sweet passion: You slide on to the floor when she's tired.
Wild passion: You oil your bodies first to ensure a slick ride.

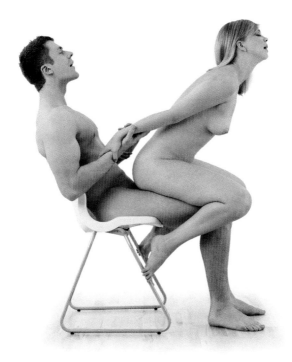

Tonight: He pulls her on to his lap, and prepares her for take-off.

Clean passion: He makes her feel secure with his powerful wrist grip.
Kinky passion: Wickedly, he cuffs her ankles to the chair legs.

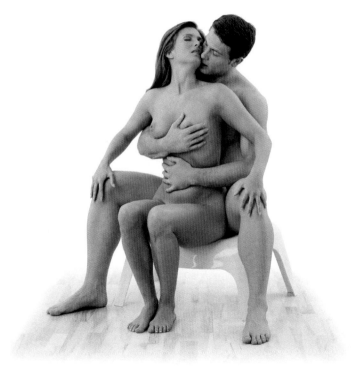

Tonight: He entices her into his study for a night of lap love.

Fun passion: He says: "Something important came up."
Fervent passion: He says: "I want you… now."

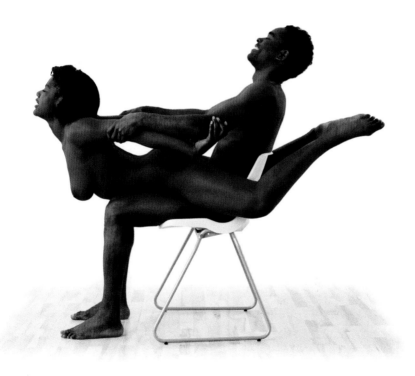

Tonight: He pops his joystick in, and makes her feel like she's flying.

Sweet passion: He holds her firmly on his cockpit.
Wild passion: She loses control, and has a glorious crash landing.

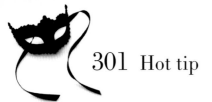

301 Hot tip

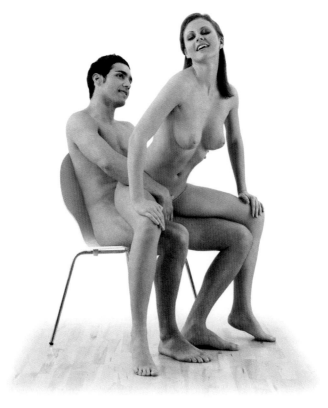

Tonight: She lowers herself on to his tip as part of a teasing lap dance.

Quickie passion: She stays to gyrate on his tip.
Lingering passion: She moves off to tease him some more.

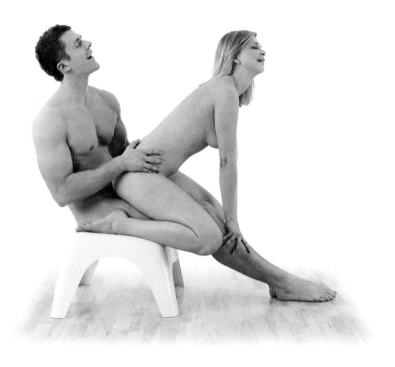

Tonight: She kneels astride him, and he eases her back on his nozzle.

Fun passion: She asks for a full tank.
Fervent passion: He grips her tight when his fuel flows.

303 Bawdy boardroom

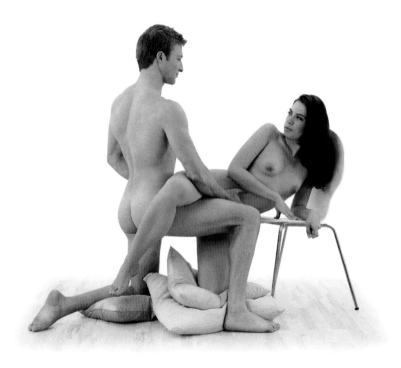

Tonight: You give each other executive relief on the boardroom floor.

Quickie passion: You've got a ten-minute window in your schedule.
Lingering passion: You cancel all meetings and close the blinds.

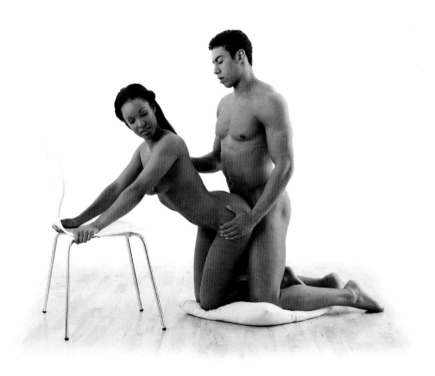

Tonight: You enjoy after-hours friskiness with the aid of an office chair.

Fun passion: He says: "I've got some urgent dick-tation for you."
Fervent passion: He buries his face in her neck, and you move in synchrony.

305 Private gym session

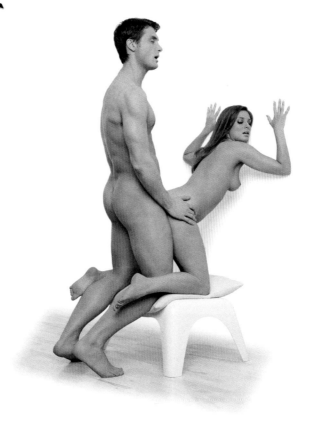

Tonight: You've finished a workout, and the gym is yours for the night...

Clean passion: She kneels on a bench while he towels her down.
Kinky passion: She kneels on a bench while he takes her against the wall.

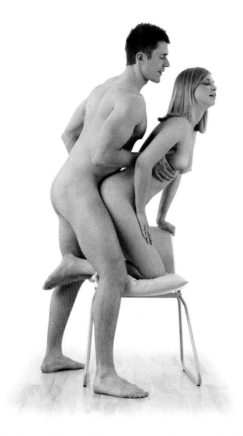

Tonight: He takes her on a chair for some fast lovin'.

Beginner passion: She braces herself against a nearby wall.
Sexpert passion: She leans forward, hands on chair, and wiggles her butt.

307 Happy humpers

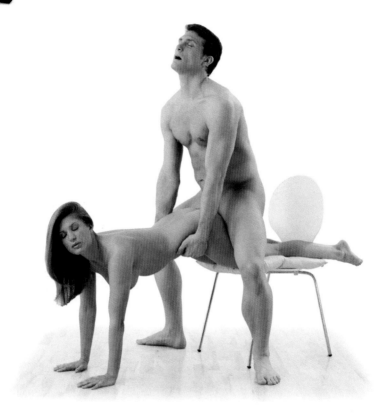

Tonight: She balances on a chair as he humps, bumps, and pumps.

Clean passion: You make sure that no one will walk in on you.
Kinky passion: Enjoy naughty fantasies about being seen.

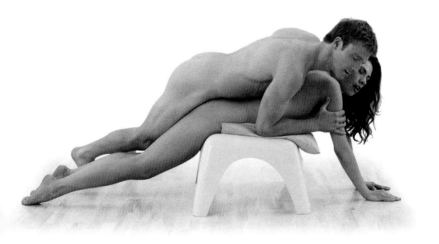

Tonight: He gives her an extra-firm vote of confidence.

Fun passion: He tells her that she has great credentials.
Fervent passion: He pushes his investment up as high as it'll go.

309 Kinky kennel

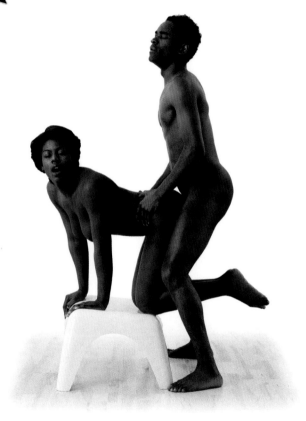

Tonight: She gets on all fours, and he pops his pooch into her kennel.

Clean passion: You cuddle up together like a pair of puppies.
Kinky passion: You dress for the occasion in dog collars and leashes.

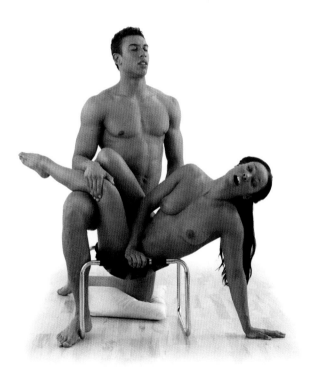

Tonight: She goes off on a tangent, and explores sideways sex-chair poses.

Beginner passion: He twists her around to align her with his main attraction.
Sexpert passion: You buy a sex swing for even more sexperimentation.

311 Fast and loose

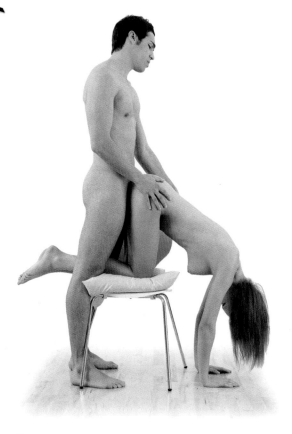

Tonight: You make it an evening of fast-thrusting, head-rush moments.

Beginner passion: He stays nice and shallow.
Sexpert passion: He goes in dirty and deep.

Ballet mistress 312

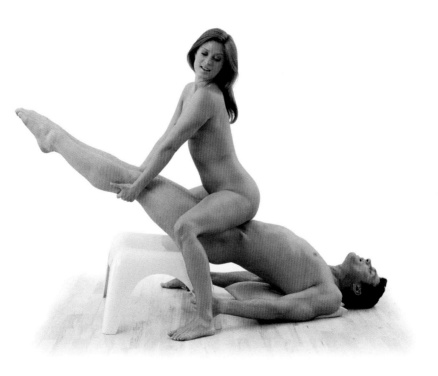

Tonight: She keeps him behind after class so she can work on his points.

Clean passion: She stands astride him, and does perfect pliés.
Kinky passion: It turns her on when he wears a tiara and a tutu.

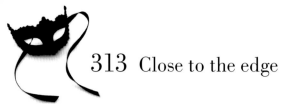

313 Close to the edge

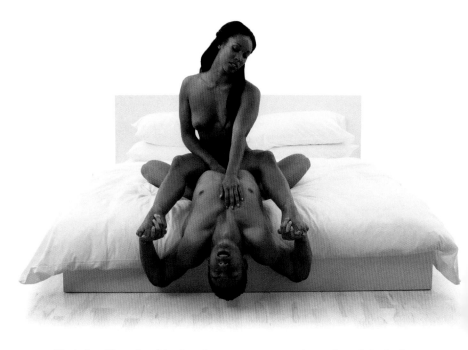

Tonight: She takes him into her core as you explore edge-of-the-bed poses.

Sweet passion: He lavishes sensual strokes on her feet.
Wild passion: She rides him so hard that she pushes him over the edge.

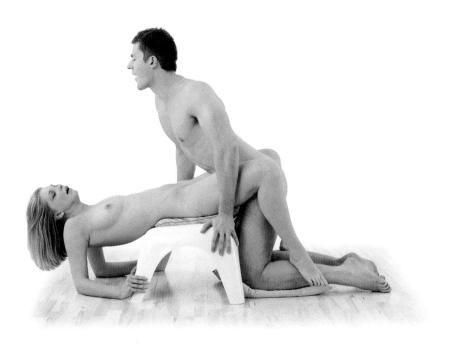

Tonight: You try out all your favorite high-impact positions.

Sweet passion: He holds her perfectly still in his arms.
Wild passion: He creates supersonic waves of pleasure as he slams into her.

315 Saucy standing orders

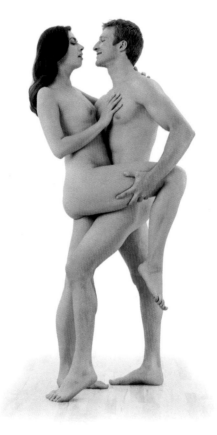

Tonight: She's the boss, and she wants him standing and erect.

Clean passion: She asks him to cover her neck in kisses.
Kinky passion: She demands that he dress in rubber, PVC, or leather.

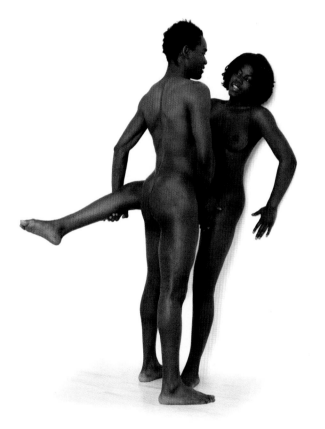

Tonight: He presses her against a wall, and feeds her fire with his hand.

Sweet passion: She uses her leg like a hook, and draws him in.
Wild passion: He lifts her up, and provokes her with his poker.

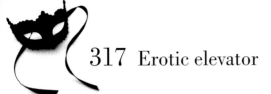

317 Erotic elevator

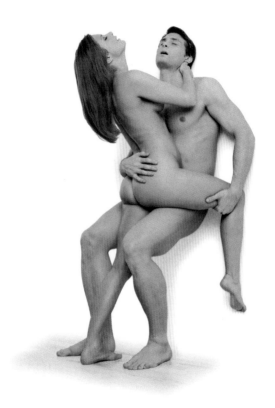

Tonight: You have wicked sex in an elevator.

Quickie passion: He presses the button that takes her straight to the top.
Lingering passion: You frolic in the basement, and kiss at every floor.

Wall hot and bothered 318

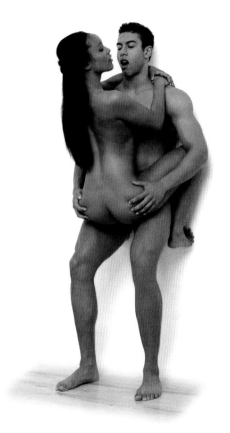

Tonight: You discover the sexy possibilities of your bedroom wall.

Sweet passion: She takes his ear lobe in her lips, and breathes in his ear.
Wild passion: You pound the wall so ferociously that you wake next door.

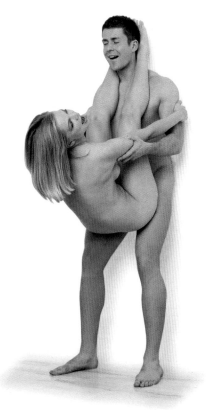

Tonight: He promises to support her in a series of mid-air maneuvers.

Sweet passion: He puts pillows on the floor just in case…
Wild passion: She leans backward into a hot handstand.

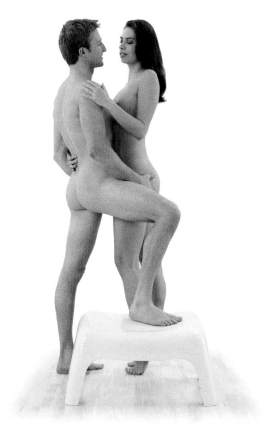

Tonight: You try every variation of standing sex.

Beginner passion: She stands on her tiptoes, and he slips inside.
Sexpert passion: He picks her up, and rocks her on his rod.

321 Two-legged race

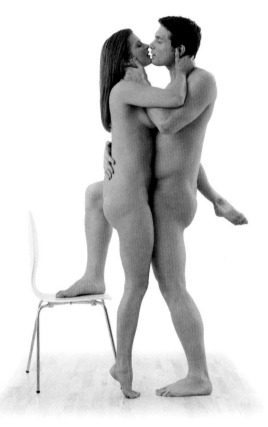

Tonight: You hold each other tight as you race towards the finish line.

Clean passion: You fall over and call it a tie.
Kinky passion: You get lost in each other's eyes, and forget who wins.

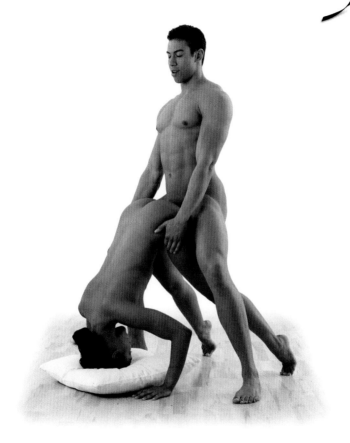

Tonight: He scales her slopes, and enters her crevices.

Quickie passion: You slam against each other for a speedy ascent.
Lingering passion: He takes his ice ax in hand, and twirls it against her.

323 Erotic opportunist

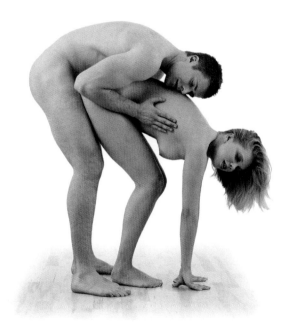

Tonight: She bends over, and he takes the chance to launch his seduction.

Quickie passion: Before she knows what's coming, her panties are down.
Lingering passion: He trails sexy kisses along the length of her spine.

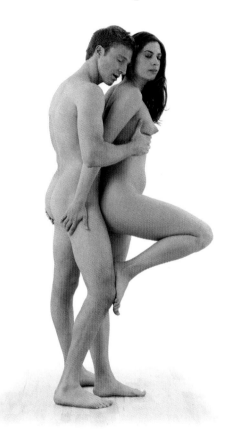

Tonight: He slinks up behind her, and gives her an urge surge.

Fun passion: He says: "Get your coat, you got lucky."
Fervent passion: He begs her to spend the night with him.

325 Double dipping

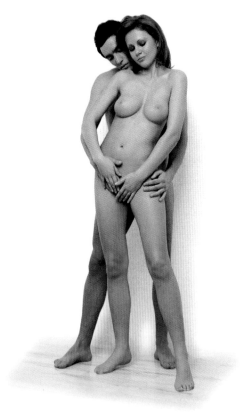

Tonight: Do it standing: he takes her from behind; she handles her front.

Clean passion: You do it sensually against the bedroom wall.
Kinky passion: You do it furtively in a public place.

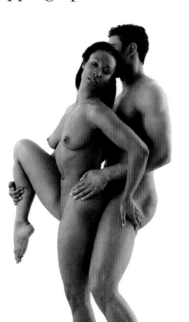

Tonight: You do some titillating teamwork to find the perfect angle.

Quickie passion: You do it in any small space.
Lingering passion: You move steamily from standing, to sitting, to lying.

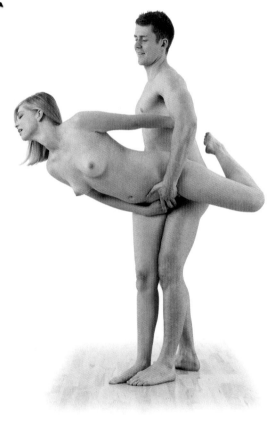

327 Love on ice

Tonight: You make love like a pair of world-class figure skaters.

Clean passion: Impress each other with your taut, lithe moves.
Kinky passion: Film yourselves, then get frisky during the playback.

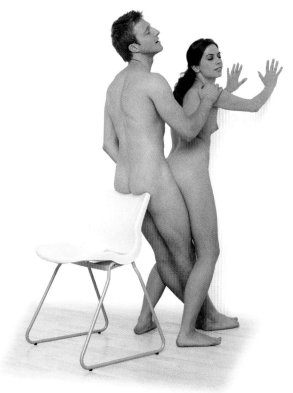

Tonight: He traps her between a wall and a hard place.

Clean passion: She takes the easy way out.
Kinky passion: He dictates the conditions of her release.

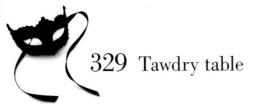

329 Tawdry table

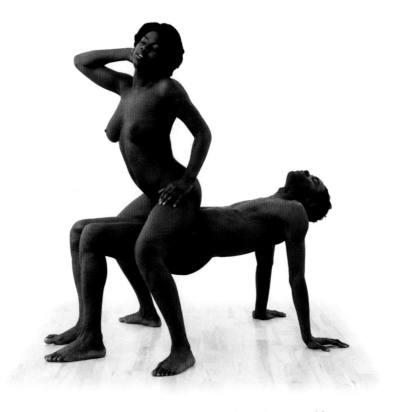

Tonight: She swirls her hips seductively on his taut tabletop.

Fun passion: She moves like she's spinning a hula-hoop.
Fervent passion: She makes him buckle with arousal.

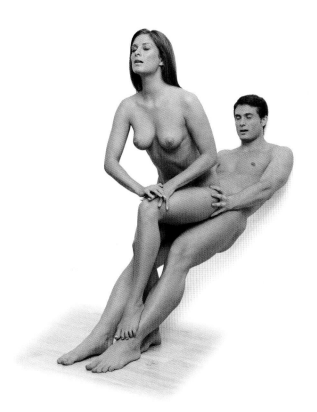

Tonight: You move your game off the green felt.

Clean passion: She feels the smoothness of his balls.
Kinky passion: He sinks her 8-ball with some hard cue action.

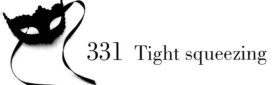

331 Tight squeezing

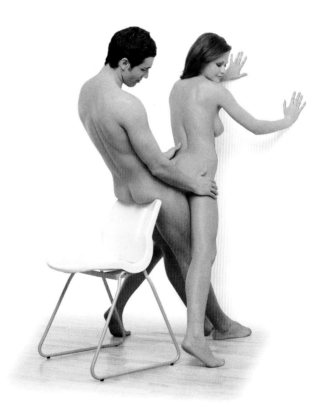

Tonight: Make it an evening of nooky in narrow spaces.

Beginner passion: You try it in the foyer before you go out.
Sexpert passion: You do it in the restaurant restroom after dessert.

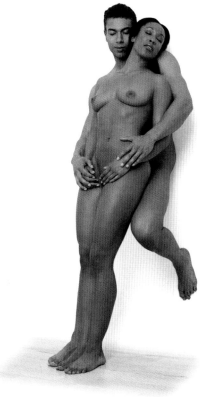

Tonight: He provides the sexy backdrop in a quiet, sensual moment.

Clean passion: You make each other shiver with some sensual stroking.
  Kinky passion: He bends her over because he's going in deep.

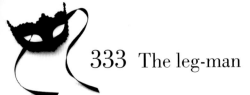

333 The leg-man

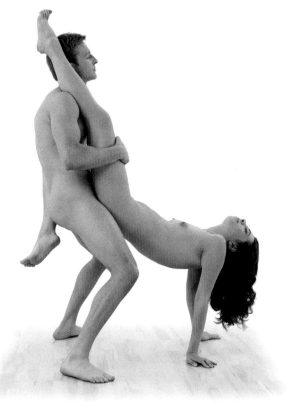

Tonight: He keeps her legs close to his heart all night long.

Beginner passion: He keeps her secure by holding her legs together.
Sexpert passion: He makes his heart murmur by parting her thighs.

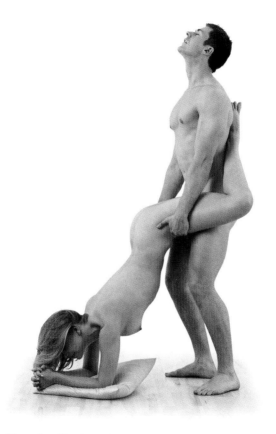

Tonight: He shows her how he moves a vacuum cleaner.

Sweet passion: He adopts a slow and steady rhythm.
Wild passion: She comes down and demonstrates her suction power.

335 All around the house

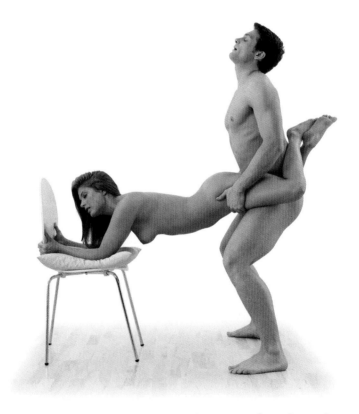

Tonight: You use the furniture to explore new angles to lovemaking.

Quickie passion: You up the ante by leaving the curtains open.
Lingering passion: You take a seat between positions.

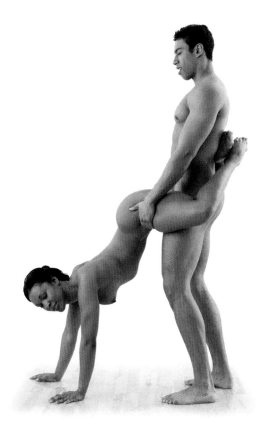

Tonight: He catches her mid-handstand, then takes amorous advantage.

Fun passion: You make this the first event in an evening of hot gymnastics.
Fervent passion: He tells her how much he adores the view.

337 Sizzling somersaults

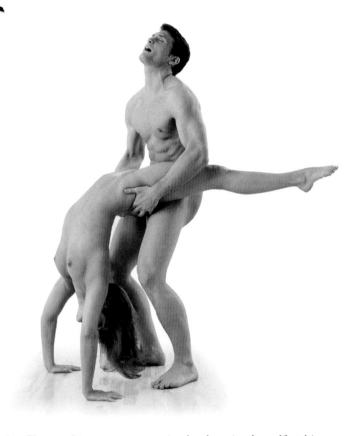

Tonight: She gets his amorous attention by throwing herself at him.

Beginner passion: He picks her up, and she does a backbend.
Sexpert passion: She makes her landing with G-spot-on precision.

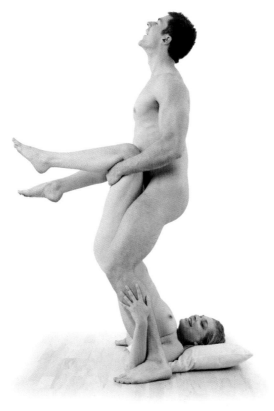

Tonight: He warms up by plunging his member between her hot thighs.

Sweet passion: He sucks her toes at the same time.
Wild passion: He drips oils on to her thighs, then moves like a dynamo.

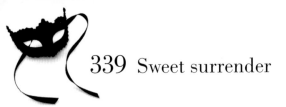

339 Sweet surrender

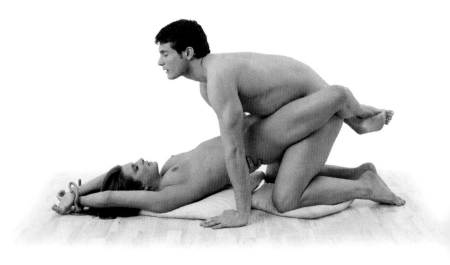

Tonight: She lies back with bound wrists, and says "Take me."

Quickie passion: He takes her instantly.
Lingering passion: He teases her by slipping in, then out again.

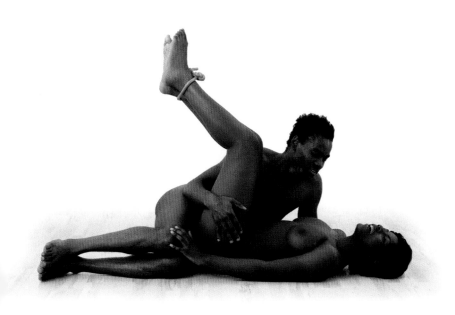

Tonight: He puts her ankles in a neat bind, then bends her to his will.

Beginner passion: She starts and finishes on her back.
Sexpert passion: She starts on her back, and finishes on all fours.

341 Happy clamping

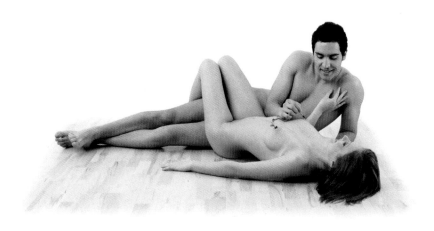

Tonight: You multiply the thrills with penetration plus clamping.

Clean passion: He lies back, and lets her move how she wants.
Kinky passion: He pops a clitoral clamp on her too.

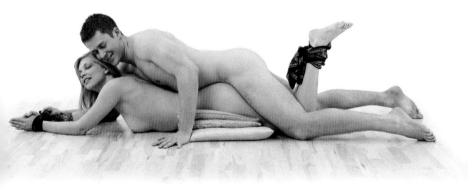

Tonight: He ties her up, then impresses her with his depth.

Clean passion: He makes it effortless for her to escape.
Kinky passion: He uses rope and bondage tape instead of scarves.

343 Lady in red

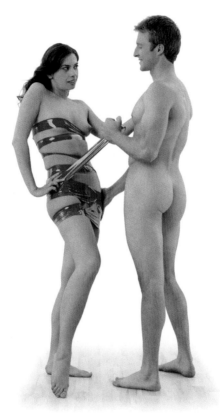

Tonight: He begins a fantasy evening by dressing her in bondage tape.

Clean passion: He covers her bits and keeps her decent.
Kinky passion: He makes a naughty access hole at the back.

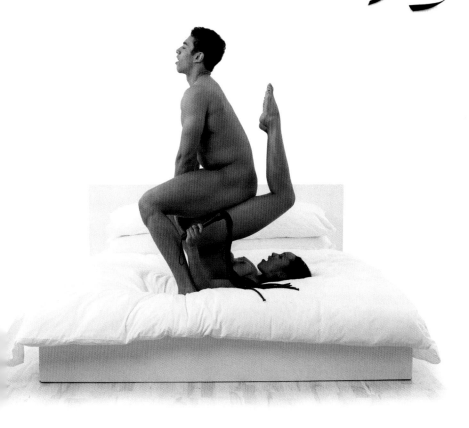

Tonight: She offers him a seat, and warns him not to be naughty.

Beginner passion: She flicks her whip on the bed.
Sexpert passion: She flicks her whip on his back.

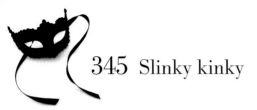

345 Slinky kinky

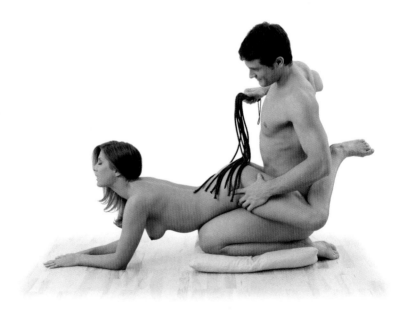

Tonight: You mix the slinkiest sex positions with the kinkiest props.

Quickie passion: Sensation overload takes you straight to orgasm.
Lingering passion: He trails his whip softly over her buttocks.

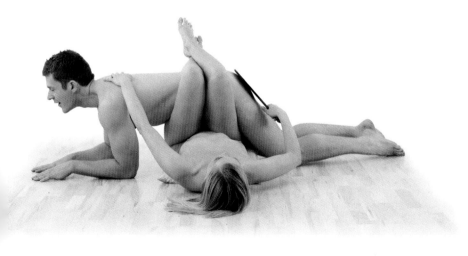

Tonight: She takes him in deep, then uses a spank paddle to make him yelp.

Beginner passion: She taps him, then rubs him better.
Sexpert passion: She whacks him until he barks.

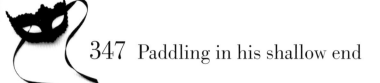

347 Paddling in his shallow end

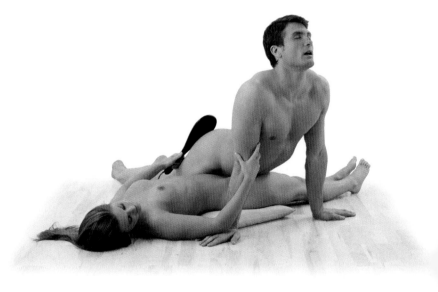

Tonight: She thwacks him with a paddle while he makes love to her.

Clean passion: She times her thwacks to his thrusts.
Kinky passion: She uses the paddle to make him go faster.

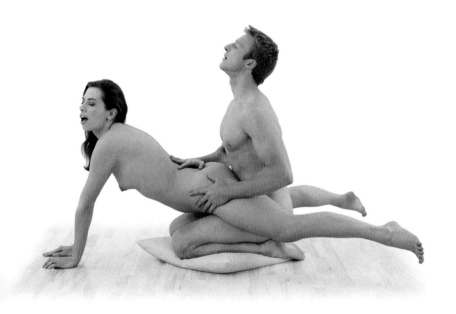

Tonight: He makes her scream by spanking and thrusting at the same time.

Fun passion: She says "Thank you" after each spank.
Fervent passion: He soothes her crimson cheeks with crushed ice.

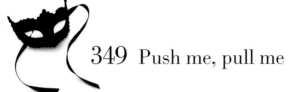

349 Push me, pull me

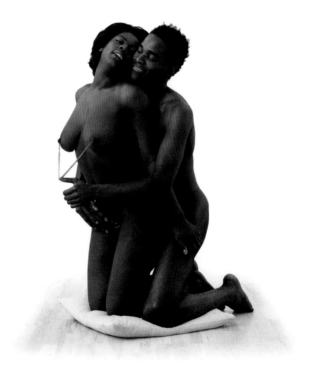

Tonight: He pushes in from behind, and pulls out from in front.

Clean passion: He asks: "How hard?"
Kinky passion: She shouts: "Don't stop!"

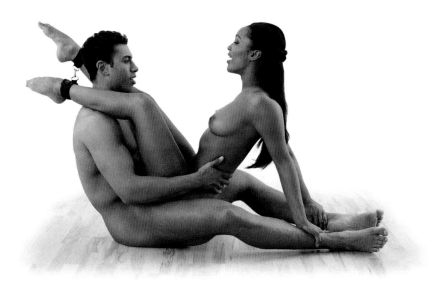

Tonight: He cuffs her ankles, and arranges her to his liking.

Fun passion: He puts her in an erotic position, and challenges her to escape.
Fervent passion: He clasps his hands behind her, and pulls her close.

351 Harnessing his hot spot

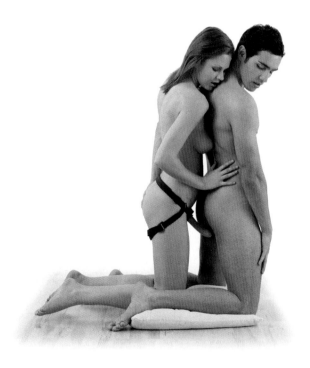

Tonight: You swap roles: she takes him with a strap-on.

Beginner passion: She slowly slips her end in.
Sexpert passion: She aims for his prostate, and brings him to the floor.

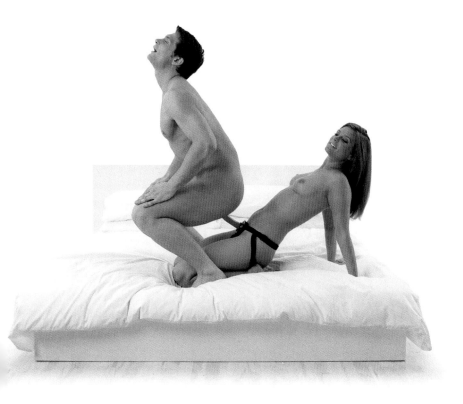

Tonight: She kneels back, and lets him go as far as he wants.

Sweet passion: She offers sexy words from behind.
Wild passion: He discovers the incendiary joy of squat thrusts.

353 Nipple naughtiness

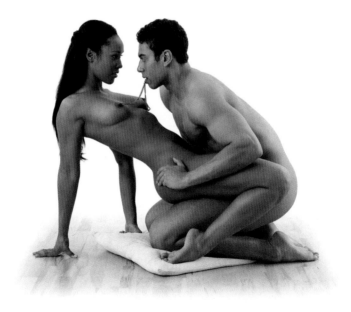

Tonight: He clamps her nipples and pulls her chain.

Quickie passion: He pulls the chain taut while she rides him mercilessly.
Lingering passion: He frees her nipples, soothes them, then clamps her again.

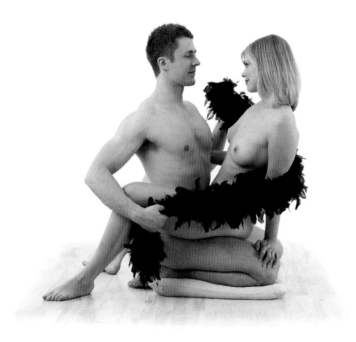

Tonight: He pulls her close for an evening of feathery pleasures.

Clean passion: He tickles her skin, and gives her goosebumps.
Kinky passion: He blindfolds her with the boa, then loses all restraint.

355 Dominatrix night

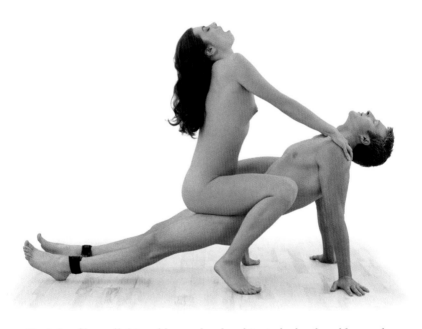

Tonight: She cuffs his ankles, and orders him to be her humble sex slave.

Quickie passion: She puts a blindfold on him, and takes him by storm.
Lingering passion: She makes him crawl helplessly around the floor.

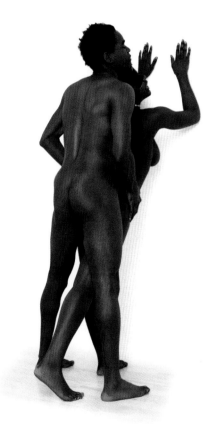

Tonight: He blindfolds her, and pins her provocatively to the wall.

   Clean passion: He slides his hands over her cutest curves.
   Kinky passion: He lets her feel the firmness of his nightstick.

357 Slave school

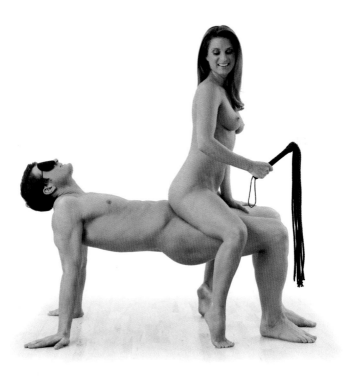

Tonight: She gives him a kinky lesson on slave etiquette.

Fun passion: If he doesn't provide a rigid seat, he gets punished.
Fervent passion: She's so overcome with lust that she drops her whip.

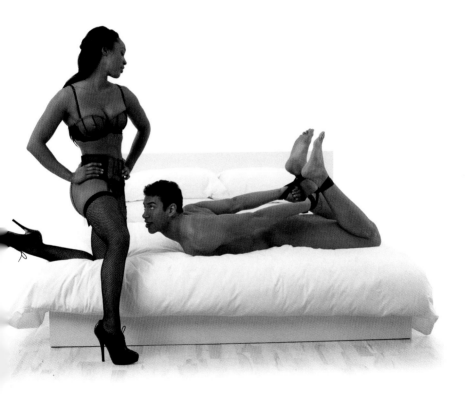

Tonight: She subjects him to erotic torture—he can look, but not touch.

Sweet passion: At the end, she massages his wrists and ankles.
Wild passion: She brings herself to a climax, just inches away from him.

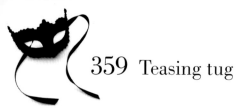

359 Teasing tug

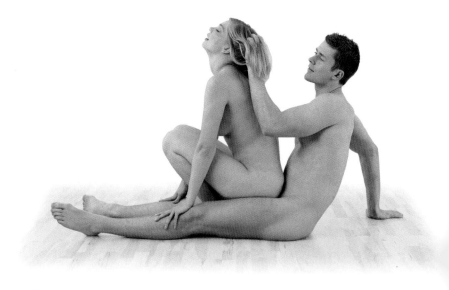

Tonight: You play around with erotic pain and try mid-coital tress-tugging.

Beginner passion: He holds her hair in a loose fist.
Sexpert passion: He holds her hair tightly because he knows her pain limits.

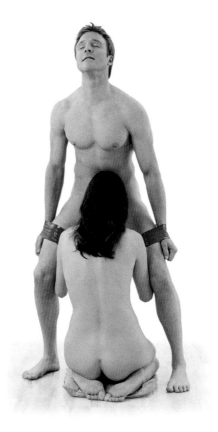

Tonight: She straps his wrists to his thighs, then gives him glorious head.

Fun passion: He must ask her permission to come.
Fervent passion: She savors the experience, and swallows him whole.

361 Dominatrix experience

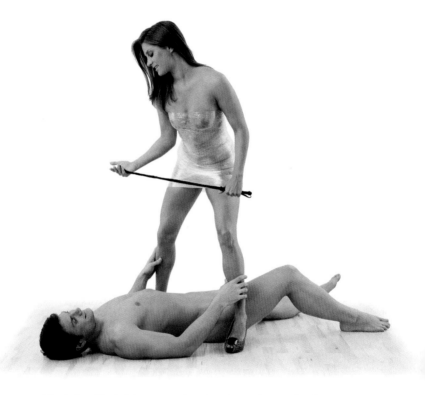

Tonight: She's his stern, whip-bearing mistress for the evening.

Sweet passion: She kisses him tenderly at the end of the night.
Wild passion: She forces him to enact her most depraved wishes.

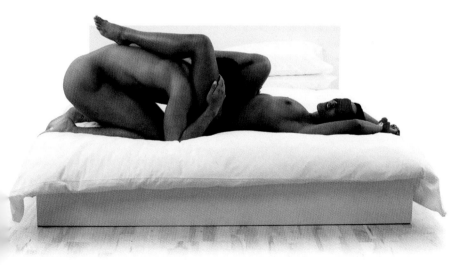

Tonight: He binds and blindfolds her, then offers his services.

Clean passion: He nuzzles and nibbles her sensitive inner thighs.
Kinky passion: He follows only her filthiest instructions.

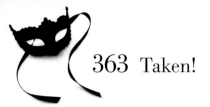

363 Taken!

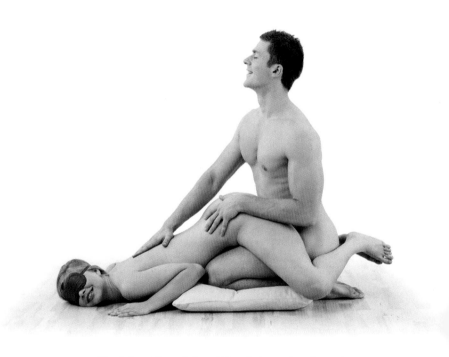

Tonight: He satisfies all her being-taken fantasies.

Clean passion: He makes her swoon as he swirls his hands over her body.
Kinky passion: You pretend that you've never met each other before.

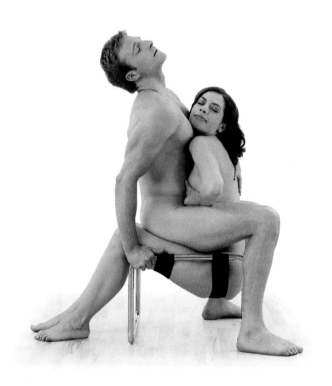

Tonight: She provides an explosive evening of massage-by-breast.

Quickie passion: She jiggles her flesh fast on his shaft.
Lingering passion: She gently teases him with her nipples.

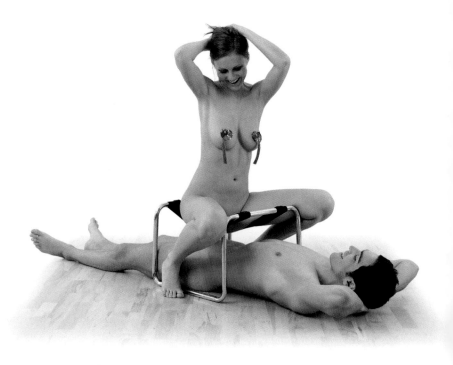

Tonight: She surprises him with a sex party for two.

Sweet passion: She says: "Don't open your eyes until I'm on top."
Wild passion: She bounces so fast that her tassels twirl.

Now it's time to start
all over again...

365 passion kit

Here's a whirlwind tour of the props, toys, and accessories that will make you gasp and moan over the coming year.

Vibrators

Battery- or AC-powered devices that deliver orgasmic vibrations—usually held against the clitoris, or inserted into the vagina, but can be used creatively on any body part.

Hot tip: Vibrators don't have to be penis-shaped. Pick the one that most tickles your fancy. Choose from lipsticks, bullets, pebbles, and even rubber ducks.

Dildos

Phallic-shaped objects—like vibrators but without the vibrations—designed to be pushed in and out of the vagina or anus.

Hot tip: For the ultimate in smoothness and style, choose a dildo made of glass.

Love eggs

Two balls or "eggs"—often attached to a cord—designed to go inside her vagina and give her a sexy full feeling. Wear these all day to build up the mood for evening.

Hot tip: Guys—pop the balls inside her before you go down on her.

G-spot toys

Insertable toys that reach the spot other sex toys don't—a specially angled tip delivers pressure and friction to her G-spot.

Hot tip: Guys—get a mental roadmap by exploring her G-spot with your fingers first.

Penis rings

A ring that sits on the base of his erect shaft—traditionally used to give him a strong erection, but often now used to give her an extra blast of clitoral stimulation during sex—thanks to the vibrator that protrudes from the ring.

Hot tip: Experiment by twisting the ring around so the vibrating attachment targets his balls.

Butt plugs

Designed for backdoor insertion, butt plugs fill up and stimulate this ultra sensitive area. Choose from textured, smooth, or vibrating butt plugs, but check that the base is flared so there's no danger of the plug doing a disappearing act.

Hot tip: Put a big dollop of lube on your lover's anus and begin with a fingertip massage.

Anal beads

A string of beads that start small and get bigger—designed to be pushed into the anal opening to give full-on sexy sensations.

Hot tip: Gently pull the beads out one by one as your lover gets near the point of no return.

Nipple clamps

Clip- or peg-like devices designed to apply sexy pressure to each nipple. Great for kinky role play.

Hot tip: Add an extra buzz—choose nipple clamps that vibrate as well as squeeze.

Handcuffs

An essential part of any bondage kit. Avoid anything with a lock and key, and choose from the friendlier Velcro, buckle, or clip options.

Hot tip: Handcuff your lover and take them repeatedly to the brink of orgasm.

Paddles

A must-have for those who love a well-aimed spank. Paddles can deliver a sensational sting or a comforting rub—some have fur on one side and rubber on the other.

Hot tip: Go for the classic spanking position—your lover on hands and knees looking penitent.

Whips

An essential tool for kinky play. Choose a whip to suit your sexual personality—anything from black leather straps to soft pink tassels.

Hot tip: Use the whip to deliver sexy psychological thrills rather than hard-core pain.

Bondage tape

This makes erotic tying up easy. There are no knots to master—you simply bind your partner with tape that sticks to itself, rather than to skin (which means that the tape removal won't hurt).

Hot tip: Start with simple wrist tying before tying your lover on to chairs/beds etc.

Dressing-up box

No kit is complete without sexy costumes—whether it's a captain's hat, a thong, or a red wig, transform your sexual personality in seconds!

Hot tip: Make your lover's day—open the door dressed in something completely outrageous.

Feathers

Whether it's a feather duster or a feather boa, feathers can drive your lover to the heights of sensuality.

Hot tip: Glide a feather from the nape of your lover's neck to the curve of their buttocks.

Massage oil

Glide your way through the night with the help of some gorgeously slippery massage oil. Just one caution: oil can damage condoms.

Hot tip: Rub oil into each other's bodies until you both shine.

Sexy food

Make sex sumptuous and decadent with erotic food. Include these on your shopping list: cream, strawberries, raspberries, passion fruit, figs, mango, ice-cream, honey…

Hot tip: Get really messy and then share a hot shower afterward.

PUBLISHER'S NOTE:
Neither the publisher nor the author is engaged in rendering professional advice or services to the individual reader, and neither shall be liable or responsible for any loss or damage allegedly arising from any information or suggestion in this book. All participants in such activities must assume the responsibility for their own actions and safety and for compliance with all applicable laws. If you have any health problem or any medical condition, or any other concerns about whether you are able to participate in any of these activities, you should take the appropriate precautions. The information contained in this book cannot replace professional advice or sound judgment and good decision making, nor does the scope of this book allow for the disclosure of all the potential hazards and risks involved in such activities.

DK would like to thank John Rowley (photographer), Gianni Mosella (assistant to photographer), Kat Mead (photography direction), Peter Mallory (photography production), and Enzo Volpe (hair and make-up). Thank you to Clare Hubbard for proofreading and Tom Howells for editorial assistance.

Special thanks to Kesta Desmond.